ADVANCES IN HOST DEFENSE MECHANISMS
Volume 7

MOLECULAR ASPECTS OF IMMUNE RESPONSE
AND INFECTIOUS DISEASES

ADVANCES IN HOST DEFENSE MECHANISMS

Series Editors

John I. Gallin, *Bethesda, Maryland*
Anthony S. Fauci, *Bethesda, Maryland*

Editorial Advisory Board

Advances in Host Defense Mechanisms

Volume 7

Molecular Aspects of Immune Response and Infectious Diseases

H. Kiyono, D.D.S., Ph.D.

Department of Oral Biology
The University of Alabama
at Birmingham
UAB Station
Birmingham, Alabama 35294

E. Jirillo, M.D.

Immunologia
Facolta di Medicina e Chirurgia
Universita di Bari
Bari, Italy 70100

C. DeSimone, M.D.

Malattie Infettive
Facolta di Medicina e Chirurgia
Universita degli Studie dell'Aquilla degli Abruzzi
L'Aquilla, Italy 67100

Raven Press ✒ New York

Raven Press, 1185 Avenue of the Americas, New York, New York 10036

Made in the United States of America

Library of Congress Cataloging-in-Publication Data

Molecular aspects of immune response and infectious diseases / [edited by] Hiroshi Kiyono, Emilio Jirillo, Claudio DeSimone.
    p.   cm. — (Advances in host defense mechanisms ; v. 7)
    Proceedings of the International Conference on Molecular Aspects of Immune Response and Infectious Diseases, held in Rome July 25–28, 1989.
    Includes bibliographical references.
    Includes index.
    ISBN 0-88167-686-1
    1. Communicable diseases—Immunological aspects—Congresses.   2. Cellular immunity--Congresses.   3. Interleukins—Congresses.   4. T cells—Receptors—Congresses.
5. Lymphocytes—Congresses.   I. Kiyono, Hiroshi.   II. Jirillo, Emilio.   III. De Simone, Claudio.   IV. International Conference on Molecular Aspects of Immune Response and Infectious Diseases (1989 : Rome, Italy)   V. Series. [DNLM: 1. Communicable Diseases--immunology—congresses.   2. Immunity, Cellular—physiology—congresses.
3. Lymphocytes—physiology—congresses.   4. Receptors. Interleukin-2—immunology--congresses.   W1 AD636 v. 7 / QW 568 M7177 1989]
RC112.M65   1990
616.9 '0479—dc20
DNLM/DLC
for Library of Congress   90-8843
                                                                                                                      CIP

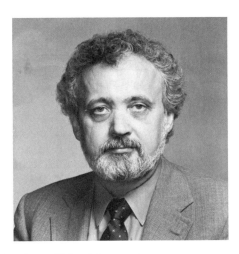

Edwin H. Beachey (1934 - 1989)

Dr. Edwin H. Beachey, who made major scientific contributions to the field of Infectious Diseases and Immunology, passed away on October 27, 1989 in Memphis, Tennessee while this book was in press. He was 55 years old. The onset of his illness prevented him from attending the International Conference on Molecular Aspects of Immune Response and Infectious Diseases, at which he was to deliver the paper included in this Proceeding.

Born in Arthur, Illinois, Dr. Beachey received a degree in chemistry from Goshen College in 1958 and his M.D. degree from Northwestern University Medical School in 1962. During medical school he developed acute rheumatic fever, a recurrence of the disease he had suffered as a boy, and came under the care and scientific tutelage of Dr. Gene Stollerman, a leading streptococcal investigator who recognized his talent and encouraged him to pursue medical research. After more training in Chicago and a research fellowship at the NIH, he rejoined Dr. Stollerman in Memphis in 1966, where they established what became an internationally recognized center for the study of the biology and pathogenesis of group A streptococci.

At the time of his death, Dr. Beachey was Professor of Medicine and Microbiology, and Chief of the Division of Infectious Diseases at the University of Tennessee College of Medicine. He was also Associate Chief of Staff for Research and Development and Director of the Infectious Disease Research Program at the Memphis Veterans Administration Medical Center. Because of his remarkable ability to recruit and train gifted investigators, he was mentor to over 70 students and postdoctoral fellows, several of whom have gone on to outstanding careers.

Dr. Beachey's twenty-three year search to understand the chemistry and immunology of streptococcal M protein led him to become one of the world's foremost scholars of bacterial pathogenesis. In many aspects his original approach to unravelling the molecular mechanisms of microbial pathogenesis using protein structural analysis and recombinant DNA technology became the dogma for many investigators and students in tackling scientific problems. He was at the forefront of the innovative use of synthetic peptides to develop models of pathogenesis and open new approaches to vaccine development. In addition, he pioneered in the field of bacterial adherence, with milestone observations involving both Gram-positive and Gram-negative bacteria. At the time he initiated his brilliant studies together with his colleague and friend Dr. Itzhak Ofek, very little was known on the molecular basis of this phenomenon nor was there any evidence to support its importance in infections. His research efforts yielded important discoveries with generic implications that went beyond the scope of bacterial pathogenesis, earning him international scientific recognition. A scientist of impeccable scientific recognition and standards, he authored or coauthored over 200 publications, including some 170 original papers, as well as books and book chapters, and had several patents to his credit.

A commitment to service kept Dr. Beachey busy as a reviewer and editor for many peer-review journals, serving numerous granting agencies, as well as the FDA, WHO, NSF and others. He delivered countless lectures and chaired many symposia around the world. His research brought him a host of prestigious awards and honors, including one of the first NIH MERIT awards, and election to numerous distinguished research societies. He died on the day he was to be informed he had won the William S. Middleton Award, the U.S. Veterans Administration's highest scientific honor for medical research.

Ed Beachey was a modest man who gave freely and generously of himself, and shared his ideas and science with others. He had an unusually wide international circle of scientific collaborators and acquaintances, several of whom counted Ed and his lovely wife Carol as intimate friends and journeyed to Memphis to enjoy the lively discussions and warmth of their home.

Dr. Beachey's diverse breadth of knowledge, familiarity with the literature and his astute insight into a wide variety of biological problems made him an invaluable source of ideas and information. Working with him was always a pleasure; he created an atmosphere of excitement around the laboratory, engaging colleagues in stimulating discussions punctuated with humor. He had the ability to initiate imaginative thinking through his encouragement and enthusiasm. Those of us fortunate enough to interact with him, to enjoy his warmth, conversation and hospitality will forever feel the pain of his loss.

At the American Society for Microbiology meeting in the spring of 1989, Dr. Beachey was officially elected to become Editor-in-Chief of *Infection and Immunity*; however, his friends sensed something was wrong. Shortly after, he was diagnosed with cancer. Throughout his illness, he was determined to continue what he enjoyed most, designing experiments, discussing science and working on manuscripts. The day before he died, he learned of new results in the laboratory confirming a hypothesis he had proposed two years earlier. It was the last time he said, "Fantastic!"

Preface

Infectious disease still remains as a major life-threatening event for mankind. Although some infectious diseases are well controlled in developed countries and most of the complications of infectious diseases are generally thought to be problems only occurring in developing areas, the appearance of new and newly-recognized infectious diseases, for example HIV-induced AIDS, have caused an increased awareness of existing infectious disease problems in all societies. This has lent a sense of urgency to understanding the host immune response to different pathogens in detail at the levels of cellular and molecular biology. Thus, recent advances in understanding the gene organization and cloned products of T-cell receptors, immunoglobulins and cytokines provide novel approaches to the new and old problems in the process of infection and host responses.

This volume contains several important new immunobiological findings concerning the precise molecular and cellular aspects of host responses to foreign antigens, including those of pathogens. We were interested in summarizing current immunological research in four major areas: the T cell receptor and antigen recognition; B cell development and immunoglobulins; cytokines and immunoregulation; and host-parasite interactions in immune diseases. Involvement of different cytokines in the development of hemopoietic stem cells into mature lymphocytes and in the specific immune response has been extensively described. The molecular characterization of individual cytokines produced by immunocytes and nonlymphoid cells, and their interaction with their respective cytokine-specific receptor-bearing immunocompetent cells is also reviewed. This volume contains new concepts of the importance of the released form of the T cell receptor (TCR) and T cell associated surface molecules for the regulation of immune responses. Further, the regulatory role of two subsets of CD4 + T cells is discussed. Recent developments in mucosal immunity and host-parasite interactions are summarized. Further, responses of the host immune system against pathogenic or auto-antigens are described in the context of several immunological diseases. Possible applications of these clinical and basic immunobiological findings to the development of effective vaccines have been emphasized.

This book will provide immunologists and infectious disease researchers with an overview of the latest research on the immune response to infectious disease at the molecular and cellular level.

EDITORS
MARCH 1990

Acknowledgments

The purpose of the International Conference on *Molecular Aspects of Immune Response and Infectious Diseases* was to provide a forum to discuss emerging aspects of modern immunobiology and their application for the understanding of infectious disease. This conference was held in Rome July 25–28, 1989. On behalf of the organizers, we appreciate very much the invited speaker's willingness to participate in this conference and to provide excellent lectures in their respective fields. We would also like to express our appreciation to the conference participants from all countries who shared their important findings and thoughts with us.

The organization of this outstanding conference and the publication of this important proceeding required cooperation and dedication from many individuals. The secretarial staffs of the conference, led by *Mr. and Mrs. Biagianti* (Travel Station, Rome), are gratefully acknowledged. *Ms. Sandra Roberts* (University of Alabama at Birmingham) and *Mr. Luciano Lucci* (University of Rome) played an important role in organizing the program of invited speakers and poster presenters. Publication of the papers would not have been possible without *Ms. Roberts'* expert skill and dedication. We would like to thank *Drs. Kerry Willis* and *Graham V. Lees* of Raven Press for providing us the opportunity to publish this proceeding. Finally, we would like to acknowledge financial support from the following: Sigma-Tau S.P.A., Italy; Smith Kline & French, Italy; Wellcome, Italy; Cilag, Italy; Sandoz, Italy; Italtarmaco, Italy; Merck, Sharp & Dohme, Italy; Becton Dickinson, Italy; Delalande, Italy; Istituto Sieroterapico Berna, Italy; Sclavo, Italy; Ellem, Italy; Glaxo, Italy; Poli Industria Chimica, Italy; Serono, Italy; Squibb, Italy; Ortho Diagnostic System, Italy; Group BSN Danone, France; Nestle, Switzerland; Beghin-Say, France; University of Alabama at Birmingham, Research Center in Oral Biology, USA (H. Birkedal-Hansen, D.D.S., Ph.D.); F. Hoffman - La Roche, Co., Switzerland (Drs. M. Steinmetz and E. Herzog); Procter and Gamble, Co., USA (R.E. Singer, Ph.D.); Bethesda Research Laboratories (M.C. Grove); Syntex Research, USA (R.N. Havemeyer, Ph.D.); Advanced Magnetics, Inc., USA (D. Vaccaro, Ph.D.). Without their appreciation for science, we could not have organized this excellent conference.

Editors
April, 1990

Contents

Lymphocyte Development

Immunological Approaches to Prevention of Infectious Diseases

To Our Families   *Momoyo and Erika*
Anna and Felicita
Alessandra and Valeria

Contributors

E. Abe, *Department of Molecular Biology, DNAX Research Institute of Molecular and Cellular Biology, Palo Alto, California 94304, USA*

B. Adkins, *Stanford University, School of Medicine, Stanford, California 94305, USA*

A. Alavi, *Department of Immunology, University College, Middlesex School of Medicine, Arthur Stanley House, 40-50 Tottenham Street, London W1P 9PG, United Kingdom*

E. Appella, *Experimental Immunology Branch, Laboratory of Cell Biology, National Cancer Institute, National Institutes of Health, Bethesda, Maryland 20892, USA*

K. Arai, *Department of Molecular Biology, The Institute of Medical Science, University of Tokyo, 4-6-1 Shirokanedai, Minato-ku, Tokyo, Japan*

N. Arai, *Department of Molecular Biology, DNAX Research Institute of Molecular and Cellular Biology, Palo Alto, California 94304, USA*

Y. Asano, *Department of Immunology, Faculty of Medicine, University of Tokyo, 7-3-1 Hongo, Bunkyo-ku, Tokyo 113, Japan*

C. Auriault, *Centre d'Immunologie et de Biologie Parasitaire, Unité Mixte INSERM U 167-CNRS 624, Institute Pasteur, 1 rue du Prof. Calmette, 59019 LILLE Cédex, France*

J. S. Axford, *Rheumatology Research, University College, Middlesex School of Medicine, Arthur Stanley House, 40-50 Tottenham Street, London W1P 9PG, United Kingdom*

J. M. Balloul, *Centre d'Immunologie et de Biologie Parasitaire, Unité Mixte INSERM U 167-CNRS 624, Institute Pasteur, 1 rue du Prof. Calmette, 59019 LILLE Cedéx, France*

E. H. Beachey, *VA Medical Center, 1030 Jefferson Avenue (151), Memphis, Tennessee 38104, USA, and University of Tennessee, 956 Court Avenue, Memphis, Tennessee 38163, USA*

K. W. Beagley, *Departments of Microbiology and Medicine, The University of Alabama at Birmingham, UAB Station, Birmingham, Alabama 35294, USA*

S. Z. Ben-Sasson, *Laboratory of Immunology, National Institute of Allergy and Infectious Diseases, National Institutes of Health, Bethesda, Maryland 20892, USA, and Lautenberg Center for Tumor Biology, Hebrew University-Hadassah Medical Center, Jerusalem, Israel*

J. Bienenstock, *Department of Pathology, Molecular Virology and Immunology Programme, Intestinal Diseases Research Unit, McMaster University, Hamilton, Ontario, Canada L8N 3Z5*

M. G. Blennerhassett, *Department of Pathology, Molecular Virology and Immunology Programme, Intestinal Diseases Research Unit, McMaster University, Hamilton, Ontario, Canada L8N 3Z5*

K. Bodman, *Department of Immunology, University College, Middlesex School of Medicine, Arthur Stanley House, 40-50 Tottenham Street, London W1P 9PG, United Kingdom*

C. A. Bona, *Department of Microbiology, Mount Sinai School of Medicine, New York, New York, USA*

A. Bond, *Department of Immunology, University College, Middlesex School of Medicine, Arthur Stanley House, 40-50 Tottenham Street, London W1P 9PG, United Kingdom*

D. Boulanger, *Centre d'Immunologie et de Biologie Parasitaire, Unité Mixte INSERM U 167–CNRS 624, Institute Pasteur, 1 rue du Prof. Calmette, 59019 LILLE Cédex, France*

P. D. Burrows, *Division of Developmental and Clinical Immunology, Department of Microbiology, University of Alabama at Birmingham, Birmingham, Alabama 35294, USA*

A. Capron, *Centre d'Immunologie et de Biologie Parasitaire, Unité Mixte INSERM U 167–CNRS 624, Institute Pasteur, 1 rue du Prof. Calmette, 59019 LILLE Cédex, France*

M. Capron, *Centre d'Immunologie et de Biologie Parasitaire, Unité Mixte INSERM U 167–CNRS 624, Institute Pasteur, 1 rue du Prof. Calmette, 59019 LILLE Cédex, France*

J. -C. Cerottini, *Ludwig Institute for Cancer Research, Lausanne Branch, 1066 Epalinges, Switzerland*

M. Chedid, *Department of Microbiology and Immunology, Wake Forest University Medical Center, 300 South Hawthorne Road, Winston-Salem, North Carolina 27103, USA*

B. Colaco, *Department of Immunology, University College, Middlesex School of Medicine, Arthur Stanley House, 40-50 Tottenham Street, London W1P 9PG, United Kingdom*

D. Conrad, *Department of Microbiology, Medical College of Virginia, Richmond, Virginia 23298, USA*

A. Cooke, *Department of Immunology, University College, Middlesex School of Medicine, Arthur Stanley House, 40-50 Tottenham Street, London W1P 9PG, United Kingdom*

M. D. Cooper, *Division of Developmental and Clinical Immunology, Departments of Microbiology, Pediatrics and Medicine, Howard Hughes Medical Institute, University of Alabama at Birmingham, Birmingham, Alabama 35294, USA*

R. M. Crawford, *Department of Cellular Immunology, Walter Reed Army Institute of Research, Washington, DC 20307-5100, USA*

K. Croitoru, *Department of Pathology, Molecular Virology and Immunology Programme, Intestinal Diseases Research Unit, McMaster University, Hamilton, Ontario, Canada L8N 3Z5*

R. de Waal Malefijt, *Department of Molecular Biology, DNAX Research Institute of Molecular and Cellular Biology, Palo Alto, California 94304, USA*

P. Delves, *Department of Immunology, University College, Middlesex School of Medicine, Arthur Stanley House, 40-50 Tottenham Street, London, W1P 9PG, United Kingdom*

R. A. Dwek, *Glycobiology Unit, Department of Biochemistry, University of Oxford, South Parks Road, Oxford, United Kingdom*

K. Eichmann, *Max-Planck-Institute für Immunbiologie, Freiburg, Federal Republic of Germany*

J. H. Eldridge, *Department of Microbiology, The University of Alabama at Birmingham, UAB Station, Birmingham, Alabama 35294, USA*

P. B. Ernst, *Department of Pathology, Molecular Virology and Immunology Programme, Intestinal Diseases Research Unit, McMaster University, Hamilton, Ontario, Canada L8N 3Z5*

F. D. Finkelman, *Department of Medicine, Uniformed Services University of the Health Sciences, Bethesda, Maryland 20814, USA*

F. W. Fitch, *The Committee on Immunology, The Department of Pathology, The Ben May Institute, University of Chicago, Box 414, 5841 South Maryland Avenue, Chicago, Illinois 60637, USA*

M. Foo-Philips, *Experimental Immunology Branch, Laboratory of Cell Biology, National Cancer Institute, National Institutes of Health, Bethesda, Maryland 20892, USA*

A. H. Fortier, *Department of Cellular Immunology, Walter Reed Army Institute of Research, Washington, DC 20307-5100, USA*

K. Fujihashi, *Department of Oral Biology, The University of Alabama at Birmingham, UAB Station, Birmingham, Alabama 35294, USA*

T. F. Gajewski, *The Committee on Immunology, The Department of Pathology, The Ben May Institute, University of Chicago, Box 414, 5841 South Maryland Avenue, Chicago, Illinois 60637, USA*

J. Gauldie, *Department of Pathology, Molecular Virology and Immunology Programme, Intestinal Diseases Research Unit, McMaster University, Hamilton, Ontario, Canada L8N 3Z5*

D. Gorman, *Department of Molecular Biology, DNAX Research Institute of Molecular and Cellular Biology, Palo Alto, California 94304, USA*

S. J. Green, *Department of Cellular Immunology, Walter Reed Army Institute of Research, Washington, DC 20307-5100, USA*

H. M. Grey, *Cytel Corporation, San Diego, California 92130, USA*

D. Grezel, *Centre d'Immunologie et de Biologie Parasitaire, Unité Mixte INSERM U 167–CNRS 624, Institute Pasteur, 1 rue du Prof. Calmette, 59019 LILLE Cédex, France*

J. M. Grzych, *Centre d'Immunologie et de Biologie Parasitaire, Unité Mixte INSERM U 167–CNRS 624, Institute Pasteur, 1 rue du Prof. Calmette, 59019 LILLE Cédex, France*

C. Guidos, *Stanford University, School of Medicine, Stanford, California 94305, USA*

R. Guy, *Experimental Immunology Branch, Laboratory of Cell Biology, National Cancer Institute, National Institutes of Health, Bethesda, Maryland 20892, USA*

K. Hatake, *Department of Molecular Biology, DNAX Research Institute of Molecular and Cellular Biology, Palo Alto, California 94304, USA*

K. S. Hathcock, *Experimental Immunology Branch, Laboratory of Cell Biology, National Cancer Institute, National Institutes of Health, Bethesda, Maryland 20892, USA*

F. C. Hay, *Department of Rheumatology Research, University College, Middlesex School of Medicine, Arthur Stanley House, 40-50 Tottenham Street, London W1P 9PG, United Kingdom*

K. Hayashida, *Department of Molecular Biology, DNAX Research Institute of Molecular and Cellular Biology, Palo Alto, California 94304, USA*

T. Heike, *Department of Molecular Biology, DNAX Research Institute of Molecular and Cellular Biology, Palo Alto, California 94304, USA*

S. Heimfeld, *Stanford University, School of Medicine, Stanford, California 94305, USA*

M. Hibi, *Institute for Molecular Biology and Cellular Biology, Osaka University, Suita, Osaka, 565 Japan*

T. Hirano, *Division of Immunology, Institute for Molecular Biology and Cellular Biology, Osaka University, Suita, Osaka, 565 Japan*

Y. Hirata, *Division of Immunology, Institute for Molecular Biology and Cellular Biology, Osaka University, Suita, Osaka, 565 Japan*

R. J. Hodes, *Experimental Immunology Branch, Laboratory of Cell Biology, National Cancer Institute, National Institutes of Health, Bethesda, Maryland 20892, USA*

T. Honjo, *The Department of Medical Chemistry, Faculty of Medicine, Kyoto University, Kyoto 606, Japan*

D. L. Hoover, *Department of Cellular Immunology, Walter Reed Army Institute of Research, Washington, DC 20307-5100, USA*

K. Inaba, *Department of Zoology, Faculty of Science, Kyoto University, Kyoto 606, Japan*

D. A. Isenberg, *Department of Rheumatology Research, University College, Middlesex School of Medicine, Arthur Stanley House, 40-50 Tottenham Street, London W1P 9PG, United Kingdom*

K. Ishizaka, *The Johns Hopkins University, School of Medicine, Baltimore, Maryland 21239*

Na. Ito, *Department of Molecular Biology, DNAX Research Institute of Molecular and Cellular Biology, Palo Alto, California 94304, USA*

No. Ito, *Department of Molecular Biology, DNAX Research Institute of Molecular and Cellular Biology, Palo Alto, California 94304, USA*

M. Iwata, *The Johns Hopkins University, School of Medicine, Baltimore, Maryland 21239*

M. Jordana, *Department of Pathology, Molecular Virology and Immunology Programme, Intestinal Diseases Research Unit, McMaster University, Hamilton, Ontario, Canada L8N 3Z5*

H. Kaneshima, *Stanford University, School of Medicine, Stanford, California 94305, USA*

K. Katamura, *The Johns Hopkins University, School of Medicine, Baltimore, Maryland 21239*

T. Kinashi, *The Department of Medical Chemistry, Faculty of Medicine, Kyoto University, Kyoto 606, Japan*

H. Kishimoto, *Department of Immunology, Faculty of Medicine, University of Tokyo, 7-3-1 Hongo, Bunkyo-ku, Tokyo 113, Japan*

T. Kishimoto, *Division of Immunology, Institute for Molecular Biology and Cellular Biology, Osaka University, Suita, Osaka, 565 Japan*

T. Kitamura, *Department of Molecular Biology, DNAX Research Institute of Molecular and Cellular Biology, Palo Alto, California 94304, USA*

H. Kiyono, *Department of Oral Biology, The University of Alabama at Birmingham, UAB Station, Birmingham, Alabama 35294, USA*

T. Komuro, *Department of Immunology, Faculty of Medicine, University of Tokyo, 7-3-1 Hongo, Bunkyo-ku, Tokyo 113, Japan*

M. Kotb, *VA Medical Center, 1030 Jefferson Avenue (151), Memphis, Tennessee 38104, USA, and University of Tennessee, 956 Court Avenue, Memphis, Tennessee 38163, USA*

R. T. Kubo, *National Jewish Center Immunology, and Respiratory Medicine, Denver, Colorado 80206, USA*

G. Le Gros, *Laboratory of Immunology, National Institute of Allergy and Infectious Diseases, National Institutes of Health, Bethesda, Maryland 20892, USA*

K. H. Lee, *The Department of Medical Chemistry, Faculty of Medicine, Kyoto University, Kyoto 606, Japan*

M. Lieberman, *Stanford University, School of Medicine, Stanford, California 94305, USA*

D. L. Leiby, *Department of Cellular Immunology, Walter Reed Army Institute of Research, Washington, DC 20307-5100, USA*

C. Lue, *Department of Microbiology, The University of Alabama at Birmingham, UAB Station, Birmingham, Alabama 35294, USA*

P. M. Lydyard, *Department of Rheumatology Research, University College, Middlesex School of Medicine, Arthur Stanley House, 40-50 Tottenham Street, London W1P 9PG, United Kingdom*

L. Mackenzie, *Department of Immunology, University College, Middlesex School of Medicine, Arthur Stanley House, 40-50 Tottenham Street, London W1P 9PG, United Kingdom*

G. Majumdar, *University of Tennessee, 956 Court Avenue, Memphis, Tennessee 38163, USA*

J. S. Marshall, *Department of Pathology, Molecular Virology and Immunology Programme, Intestinal Diseases Research Unit, McMaster University, Hamilton, Ontario, Canada L8N 3Z5*

K. Maruyama, *Department of Molecular Biology, DNAX Research Institute of Molecular and Cellular Biology, Palo Alto, California 94304, USA*

J. L. Maryanski, *Ludwig Institute for Cancer Research, Lausanne Branch, 1066 Epalinges, Switzerland*

T. Matsuda, *Division of Immunology, Institute for Molecular Biology and Cellular Biology, Osaka University, Suita, Osaka, 565 Japan*

M. McCune, *Stanford University, School of Medicine, Stanford, California 94305, USA*

J. R. McGhee, *Department of Microbiology, The University of Alabama at Birmingham, UAB Station, Birmingham, Alabama 35294, USA*

K. M. McNagny, *Division of Developmental and Clinical Immunology, Department of Microbiology, University of Alabama at Birmingham, Birmingham, Alabama 35294, USA*

M. S. Meltzer, *Department of Cellular Immunology, Walter Reed Army Institute of Research, Washington, DC 20307-5100, USA*

J. Mestecky, *Departments of Microbiology, Oral Biology and Medicine, The University of Alabama at Birmingham, UAB Station, Birmingham, Alabama 35294, USA*

A. Miyajima, *Department of Molecular Biology, DNAX Research Institute of Molecular and Cellular Biology, Palo Alto, California 94304, USA*

S. Miyatake, *Department of Molecular Biology, DNAX Research Institute of Molecular and Cellular Biology, Palo Alto, California 94304, USA*

S. B. Mizel, *Department of Microbiology and Immunology, Wake Forest University Medical Center, 300 South Hawthorne Road, Winston-Salem, North Carolina 27103, USA*

Z. Moldoveanu, *Department of Microbiology, The University of Alabama at Birmingham, UAB Station, Birmingham, Alabama 35294, USA*

M. Muramatsu, *Department of Molecular Biology, DNAX Research Institute of Molecular and Cellular Biology, Palo Alto, California 94304, USA*

C. A. Nacy, *Department of Cellular Immunology, Walter Reed Army Institute of Research, Washington, DC 20307-5100, USA*

T. Nakayama, *Department of Immunology, Faculty of Medicine, University of Tokyo, 7-3-1 Hongo, Bunkyo-ku, Tokyo 113, Japan*

R. Namikawa, *Stanford University, School of Medicine, Stanford, California 94305, USA*

G. Nau, *The Committee on Immunology, The Department of Pathology, The Ben May Institute, University of Chicago, Box 414, 5841 South Maryland Avenue, Chicago, Illinois 60637, USA*

B. A. Nelson, *Department of Cellular Immunology, Walter Reed Army Institute of Research, Washington, DC 20307-5100, USA*

J. Ninomiya-Tsuji, *Department of Molecular Biology, DNAX Research Institute of Molecular and Cellular Biology, Palo Alto, California 94304, USA*

J. Nishida, *Department of Molecular Biology, DNAX Research Institute of Molecular and Cellular Biology, Palo Alto, California 94304, USA*

H. Ohno, *The Johns Hopkins University, School of Medicine, Baltimore, Maryland 21239*

P. Pala, *Ludwig Institute for Cancer Research, Lausanne Branch, 1066 Epalinges, Switzerland*

R. Palacios, *Basel Institute for Immunology, Basel, Switzerland*

R. B. Parekh, *Glycobiology Unit, Department of Biochemistry, University of Oxford, South Parks Road, Oxford, United Kingdom*

W. E. Paul, *Laboratory of Immunology, National Institute of Allergy and Infectious Diseases, National Institutes of Health, Bethesda, Maryland 20892, USA*

M. H. Perdue, *Department of Pathology, Molecular Virology and Immunology Programme, Intestinal Diseases Research Unit, McMaster University, Hamilton, Ontario, Canada L8N 3Z5*

R. J. Pierce, *Centre d'Immunologie et de Biologie Parasitaire, Unité Mixte INSERM U 167–CNRS 624, Institute Pasteur, 1 rue du Prof. Calmette, 59019 LILLE Cédex, France*

M. Plaut, *Department of Medicine, John Hopkins University School of Medicine, Baltimore, Maryland 21239, USA*

T. W. Rademacher, *Glycobiology Unit, Department of Biochemistry, University of Oxford, South Parks Road, Oxford, United Kingdom*

J. Radl, *TNO Institute of Experimental Gerontology, Rijiswijk, The Netherlands*

K. Rajewsky, *Institute for Genetics, University of Cologne, Weyertal 121, D-5000 Cologne 41, Federal Republic of Germany*

I. M. Roitt, *Department of Immunology, University College, Middlesex School of Medicine, Arthur Stanley House, 40-50 Tottenham Street, London W1P 9PG, United Kingdom*

G. Rook, *Department of Microbiology, University College, Middlesex School of Medicine, Arthur Stanley House, 40-50 Tottenham Street, London W1P 9PG, United Kingdom*

K. Sano, *Department of Immunology, Faculty of Medicine, University of Tokyo, 7-3-1 Hongo, Bunkyo-ku, Tokyo 113, Japan*

S. R. Schell, *The Committee on Immunology, The Department of Pathology, The Ben May Institute, University of Chicago, Box 414, 5841 South Maryland Avenue, Chicago, Illinois 60637, USA*

J. Schreurs, *Department of Molecular Biology, DNAX Research Institute of Molecular and Cellular Biology, Palo Alto, California 94304, USA*

J. L. Schulman, *Department of Microbiology, Mount Sinai School of Medicine, New York, New York, USA*

F. Shirakawa, *Department of Microbiology and Immunology, Wake Forest University Medical Center, 300 South Hawthorne Road, Winston-Salem, North Carolina 27103, USA*

J. Shlomai, *Hadassah Medical School, Kuvin Center for the Study of Infectious and Tropical Diseases, Jerusalem, Israel*

J. E. Sims, *Immunex Corporation, 51 University Street, Seattle, Washington 98101, USA*

L. Smith, *Stanford University, School of Medicine, Stanford, California 94305, USA*

M. Smith, *Department of Immunology, University College, Middlesex School of Medicine, Arthur Stanley House, 40-50 Tottenham Street, London W1P 9PG, United Kingdom*

G. Spangrude, *Stanford University, School of Medicine, Stanford, California 94305, USA*

A. M. Stanisz, *Department of Pathology, Molecular Virology and Immunology Programme, Intestinal Diseases Research Unit, McMaster University, Hamilton, Ontario, Canada L8N 3Z5*

R. H. Stead, *Department of Pathology, Molecular Virology and Immunology Programme, Intestinal Diseases Research Unit, McMaster University, Hamilton, Ontario, Canada L8N 3Z5*

S. Suematsu, *Division of Immunology, Institute for Molecular Biology and Cellular Biology, Osaka University, Suita, Osaka, 565 Japan*

K. Sugimoto, *Department of Molecular Biology, DNAX Research Institute of Molecular and Cellular Biology, Palo Alto, California 94304, USA*

N. Sumar, *Department of Immunology, University College, Middlesex School of Medicine, Arthur Stanley House, 40-50 Tottenham Street, London W1P 9PG, United Kingdom*

T. Tada, *Department of Immunology, Faculty of Medicine, University of Tokyo, 7-3-1 Hongo, Bunkyo-ku, Tokyo 113, Japan*

T. Taga, *Division of Immunology, Institute for Molecular Biology and Cellular Biology, Osaka University, Suita, Osaka, 565 Japan*

T. Taguchi, *Department of Oral Biology, The University of Alabama at Birmingham, UAB Station, Birmingham, Alabama 35294, USA*

K. Tashiro, *The Department of Medical Chemistry, Faculty of Medicine, Kyoto University, Kyoto 606, Japan*

M. Tomai, *VA Medical Center, 1030 Jefferson Avenue (151), Memphis, Tennessee 38104, USA, and University of Tennessee, 956 Court Avenue, Memphis, Tennessee 38163, USA*

K. Toyama, *The Department of Medical Chemistry, Faculty of Medicine, Kyoto University, Kyoto 606, Japan*

G. Tsoulfa, *Department of Immunology, University College, Middlesex School of Medicine, Arthur Stanley House, 40-50 Tottenham Street, London W1P 9PG, United Kingdom*

S. J. Ullrich, *Experimental Immunology Branch, Laboratory of Cell Biology, National Cancer Institute, National Institutes of Health, Bethesda, Maryland 20892, USA*

H. -M. Wang, *Department of Molecular Biology, DNAX Research Institute of Molecular and Cellular Biology, Palo Alto, California 94304, USA*

C. Warren, *Glycobiology Unit, Department of Biochemistry, University of Oxford, South Parks Road, Oxford, United Kingdom*

I. Weissman, *Stanford University, School of Medicine, Stanford, California 94305, USA*

P. A. Welch, *Division of Developmental and Clinical Immunology, Departments of Microbiology and Pediatrics, University of Alabama at Birmingham, Birmingham, Alabama 35294, USA*

I. Wolowczuk, *Centre d'Immunologie et de Biologie Parasitaire, Unité Mixte INSERM U 167–CNRS 624, Institute Pasteur, 1 rue du Prof. Calmette, 59019 LILLE Cédex, France*

Q. Wu, *Division of Developmental and Clinical Immunology, Department of Microbiology, University of Alabama at Birmingham, Birmingham, Alabama 35294, USA*

G-x. Xie, *Department of Molecular Biology, DNAX Research Institute of Molecular and Cellular Biology, Palo Alto, California 94304, USA*

K. Yamasaki, *Division of Immunology, Institute for Molecular Biology and Cellular Biology, Osaka University, Suita, Osaka, 565 Japan*

K. Yasukawa, *Division of Immunology, Institute for Molecular Biology and Cellular Biology, Osaka University, Suita, Osaka, 565 Japan*

T. Yokota, *Department of Molecular Biology, DNAX Research Institute of Molecular and Cellular Biology, Palo Alto, California 94304, USA*

Molecular Aspects of Immune Response and Infectious Diseases, edited by H. Kiyono, E. Jirillo, and C. DeSimone. Raven Press, Ltd., New York, © 1990.

1

Second Messengers In The Action of Interleukin 1

S. B. Mizel, F. Shirakawa, and M. Chedid

Department of Microbiology and Immunology, Wake Forest University Medical Center, 300 South Hawthorne Road, Winston-Salem, NC 27103, USA

INTRODUCTION

Interleukin 1 (IL-1) is a low molecular weight (17,000 dalton) immunoregulatory protein produced by stimulated macrophages as well as several other cell types. Although IL-1 was originally described as a co-mitogen for the *in vitro* proliferation of murine thymocytes (1), later studies revealed that IL-1 could also promote or enhance the maturation, proliferation and functional activation of a broad range of cell types that share a common involvement in immune or inflammatory responses. For example, IL-1 stimulates thymocyte maturation (2), antigen and mitogen-induced T cell proliferation (1, 3, 4), cytotoxic T cell activation (5), κ immunoglobulin (Ig) light chain synthesis and surface Ig expression in pre-B cells (6, 7), and B cell proliferation (8). Furthermore, IL-1 induces prostaglandin and collagenase production by human rheumatoid synovial cells (9) and fibroblasts (10-12), acute phase protein production by hepatocytes (13), bone resorption via osteoclast activation (14), fibroblast proliferation (12), and procoagulant activity in endothelial cells (15). In addition, IL-1 can induce fever in a variety of species (16).

INTRACELLULAR SECOND MESSENGERS FOR IL-1

IL-1 Receptors

Dower *et al.* (17, 18) first demonstrated the existence of a high affinity (Kd 10^{-10}M) receptor for IL-1 (IL-1R) on a spectrum on IL-1-responsive cells. Similar results were subsequently reported by other investigators (19-23). Although IL-1α and β share only 26% homology in their amino acid sequences, they bind to the same receptor with similar affinities.

After IL-1 binds to its receptor on murine T cells and fibroblasts, 50% of the surface-bound IL-1 is internalized within 1 to 2 hrs at 37°C and gradually moves through various cell compartments, eventually accumulating in nuclei (22). After 6 hrs, 35% of the internalized IL-1 is found within the nucleus. In some cell types, for example, EL 4 cells, the IL-1 remains in an intact form. Similar results were also obtained with human neutrophils (23). However, it remains to be determined how IL-1 translocates to the nucleus or if internalization of IL-1 is associated with any type of signal-transduction pathway.

IL-1 Signal-Transduction

Although PMA, a protein kinase C (PKC) activator, can mimic many of the biological effects of IL-1, IL-1 does not activate PKC nor induce its translocation in murine thymocytes, murine LBRM T lymphoma and IL-1-responsive human HSB subclones (24; White and Mizel, unpublished observations). Furthermore, PKC inhibitors have no inhibitory effect on IL-1-induced biological responses such as interleukin 2 (IL-2) receptor expression and κ Ig synthesis (24-28).

Several studies have demonstrated that IL-1 does not alter the level of free intracellular calcium nor does it modify phosphatidylinositol metabolism in LBRM cells, HSB T cell subclones, or human neutrophils (24, 26). In addition, calcium antagonists, which inhibit calcium influx or intracellular calcium distribution, and calmodulin inhibitors have no inhibitory effect on IL-1-induced IL-2 receptor expression in YT cells (27).

cAMP and IL-1 Signal-Transduction

Since YT cells, a human natural killer cell line, possess IL-1 receptors and also exhibit an increase in the expression of IL-2 receptors in response to IL-1 (29), we decided to use this cell line to probe the action of IL-1 (27). During the course of screening a variety of substances for their ability to induce IL-2 receptor expression, we found that dibutyrIL-cAMP was quite stimulatory. This observation prompted us to examine two other drugs, forskolin and aminophylline that directly activate adenylate cyclase or inhibit phosphodiesterase activity and thus elevate the intracellular level of cAMP. Both of these agents stimulated IL-2Rα expression on YT cells. PKC inhibitors, calcium ionophores, calcium antagonists, or calmodulin inhibitors had no effect on IL-1-dependent IL-2Rα expression on YT cells.

To more directly analyze the possibility that IL-1 may exert its biological actions via cAMP, we measured cAMP levels in cultures of YT cells incubated in the presence or absence of IL-1. It is important to note that a highly sensitive ^{125}I-cAMP radioimmunoassay kit was used in these experiments instead of a ^{3}H-cAMP kit which is far less sensitive. Purified recombinant human IL-1α and β as well as recombinant murine IL-1α induced a rapid and substantial increase in the intracellular level of cAMP in YT cells. The maximal level of induced cAMP was reached after approximately 10 min and declined to almost background levels by 120 min post-stimulation. Fifty percent of the maximal response was achieved with 0.04×10^{-11}M IL-1. Antibodies directed against each form of IL-1, i.e., human α or β or murine α, neutralized the ability of IL-1 to induce cAMP production. Since IL-1 induces the synthesis of prostaglandins and prostaglandins stimulate the production of cAMP, we tested if IL-1 increased cAMP levels via prostaglandins. Indomethacin had no effect on IL-1 stimulation of cAMP production, ruling out this possibility. Furthermore, the action of IL-1 on cAMP production was not blocked by the protein synthesis inhibitor, cycloheximide. Taken together, these results indicate that IL-1 influences cAMP production by a rapid, prostaglandin- and protein synthesis-independent mechanism.

Although the results with YT cells are suggestive of a direct link between IL-1-induced cAMP production and IL-1 action, it was essential to determine if IL-1 could induce cAMP production in other types of IL-1 responsive cells. We tested the following IL-1-responsive cell lines: the murine pre-B cell line, 70Z/3, the human B lymphoblastoid cell line, CESS, and Swiss 3T3 mouse fibroblasts. In all cases, IL-1 stimulated an increase in cAMP production in intact cells as well as membrane preparations. Furthermore, enhanced cAMP production was also obtained in primary cultures of murine thymocytes (27) and human rheumatoid synovial cells (30). Thus a relatively broad range of IL-1-responsive cell types produce cAMP in response to IL-1. Two other important observations were made that provided additional links between IL-1-induced cAMP and IL-1 action. If an elevation in cAMP was directly associated with the action of IL-1, then a given level of cAMP--independent of the agent used to induce cAMP production--should be associated with the same degree of biological response, for example, thymocyte proliferation, κ Ig synthesis, or IL-2Rα expression. Our results with IL-1 and forskolin--two inducers of cAMP production--clearly demonstrate such a relationship (27). For example, when YT cells were induced by a given concentration of IL-1 to produce 6 pmoles of cAMP, approximately 50% of the cells were IL-2Rα$^+$. Likewise, when murine thymocytes were induced by IL-1 or forskolin to produce 1 pmole of cAMP, the level of subsequent thymocyte proliferation was identical. These findings strongly establish a direct link between IL-1-induced cAMP accumulation and a variety of cellular responses ranging from IL-2 receptor expression to PGE production.

In line with our findings, Zhang *et al.* (31) also reported that IL-1 induces intracellular cAMP accumulation in the human fibroblast cell line, FS 4. In addition, IL-1 was shown to induce interleukin 6 (IL-6) production in FS 4 cells by a mechanism that was sensitive to inhibition by H8, an inhibitor for both protein kinase A (PKA) and PKC but not by H7, an inhibitor for PKC. Interestingly, tumor necrosis factor α (TNFα) which has a similar spectrum of biological activities to IL-1, also induced cAMP and IL-6 production in FS 4 cells. TNFα, like IL-1, also induced IL-2Rα expression (32) and cAMP production in YT cells (Shirakawa and Mizel, unpublished data).

In order to more directly examine the mechanism of IL-1-induced cAMP production, we next evaluated whether or not IL-1 could induce cAMP synthesis in isolated membrane fractions from YT cells. In the presence of IL-1, cAMP production was stimulated approximately seven-fold over control membranes incubated in the absence of IL-1. IL-1 stimulation of membrane cAMP production was strongly dependent on the presence of GTP. The dependence of IL-1-induced cAMP production in isolated membranes raised the possibility that the IL-1R might be linked to adenylate cyclase via a GTP-binding protein intermediate.

G-Binding Protein Involvement in IL-1 Signal-Transduction

In view of our observation that IL-1 stimulates cAMP production in a variety of cell types, and that cAMP analogs and cholera toxin can substitute for IL-1 in the induction of IL-1-mediated physiological responses, we examined the possibility that a GTP- or G-binding protein may serve as an intermediate in the signal transduction pathway linking the IL-1 receptor with adenylate cyclase activation (30).

As noted above, IL-1 can induce a significant increase in the frequency of surface Ig[+] 70Z/3 pre-B cells (via the induction of κ Ig light chain gene expression), IL-2Rα expression by the human natural killer cell line YT, and PGE_2 production by human rheumatoid synovial cells. Treatment of these cell types with pertussis toxin (PT) for 4 hrs prior to the addition of IL-1 markedly inhibited all of these events. Under the same conditions, PT also inhibited IL-1-stimulated cAMP production. This findings was rather surprising in view of the previously accepted notion that the adenylate cyclase-linked stimulatory G proteins were PT insensitive (33, 34). IL-1 also stimulated cAMP production in isolated membranes from YT, 70Z/3 cells, and mouse 3T3 fibroblasts. Interestingly, IL-1 alone caused only marginal stimulation of adenylate cyclase. But, when membranes were incubated with IL-1 and GTP, cAMP production was markedly enhanced. The requirement for GTP in IL-1-induced cAMP production fulfilled one of the criteria for involvement of a G protein in transmembrane signaling. Furthermore, membranes isolated from cells treated with PT exhibited a 50-80% decrease in cAMP production in response to IL-1. This observation not only demonstrated that the effect of PT in the whole cell experiments was not due to cytotoxicity, but also supported the view that a PT-sensitive, adenylate cyclase-linked stimulatory G protein was involved in the signal transduction pathway in several IL-1-responsive cell types.

We next investigated whether IL-1 could induce GTPase activity in isolated membranes from responsive cells. Our results demonstrated that IL-1 can rapidly stimulate a significant increase in GTPase activity in 70Z/3 membranes (two-fold in 15 sec). It is important to note that essentially all of the IL-1-inducible GTPase activity in isolated membranes was sensitive to a prior treatment of the membranes with PT.

In view of the possibility that the IL-1-responsive G protein might be distinct from previously described PT-sensitive G proteins, we next sought to define the size of the α subunit of this protein. When membranes from 70Z/3 cells were incubated in the presence of ^{32}P-labeled nicotinamide adenine dinucleotide (NAD) and PT, a 46 kD protein was labeled. This protein was not labeled in the absence of PT. Similar results were obtained with the murine thymoma EL 4 cell line.

Taken together, our results suggest that IL-1 binds to its cell surface receptor, activates a 46 kD pertussis toxin-sensitive G protein, which in turn stimulates adenylate cyclase activity and thus increases the intracellular level of cAMP. The question remained, however, as to how an elevation in cAMP was linked to the induction of specific gene transcription, for example, κ Ig light chains and IL-2Rα subunits.

NF-κB and IL-1-Induced Gene Activation

It is evident from a number of studies that gene transcription is under the control of specific DNA-binding proteins with specificity for unique DNA sequences in promoter and enhancer regions. Several of these proteins have been characterized and their functional activity and DNA sequence specificity assessed using a variety of methods (e.g., DNA mobility shift, methylation interference, and DNA footprinting assays). For example, DNA-binding proteins with specificity for regulatory regions associated with heavy and light chain immunoglobulin genes (35-40) have been characterized.

NF-κB, a DNA-binding protein that is activated in T and B cells in response to LPS, phorbol esters, and cytokines, exhibits specificity for the sequence 5'-GGGGACTTTCC-3' (35, 36, 38, 40) that is also found in the Human Immunodeficiency Virus long terminal region (HIV-LTR) (41), the genes for the IL-2Rα subunit (42, 43) and IL-2 (44). Sen and Baltimore (35) put forward the related hypothesis that LPS-induced kappa light chain gene expression in pre-B cells may also require the phosphorylation of NF-κB, perhaps via PKC.

In view of our earlier observations on the induction of κ Ig synthesis in the pre-B cell line, 70Z/3, by IL-1 (6) and cAMP (28, 43), we examined the possibility that IL-1 and cAMP might, like LPS, induce κ Ig expression via the activation of NF-κB.

In the first series of experiments (28), 70Z/3 cells were transfected with an expression plasmid (E⁻CAT) containing a reporter gene, chloramphenicol acetyl transferase (CAT), and a light chain promoter, or a second plasmid, EκCAT, that contains the CAT reporter gene, a light chain promoter, and a segment of the $J_κ$-$C_κ$ intron containing the κ enhancer (38). The cells were then stimulated with IL-1, cAMP, or forskolin. Independent of the stimulant, no CAT activity was detected in cells transfected with E⁻CAT. In contrast, IL-1, cAMP, and forskolin induced CAT activity in cells transfected with EκCAT. In a subsequent series of experiments, we used a DNA mobility shift assay to demonstrate the IL-1, cAMP, and forskolin could induce the appearance of active NF-κB in the nuclei of stimulated cells. This effect is independent of a requirement for protein synthesis. The adenylate cyclase inhibitor, ddAdo, as well as the protein kinase inhibitor, H8, inhibited the ability of IL-1 to induce NF-κB activation in 70Z/3 cells. In addition, PT treatment of cells prevented the induction of NF-κB by IL-1.

In a related series of experiments (43), we also examined the effect of IL-1 on NF-κB activation in the YT cell line that can be induced to express IL-2Rα subunits following incubation with IL-1 or cAMP inducers or analogs (43, 45). As with 70Z/3 cells, IL-1 induced the activation of NF-κB in YT cells by a mechanism that was protein-synthesis independent. The enhancer of the HIV-LTR has repeated κB motifs. When YT cells were transfected with an expression plasmid containing the HIV-LTR and the reporter gene, CAT, and stimulated with IL-1, cAMP analogs, or forskolin, CAT gene transcription was activated (Shirakawa and Mizel, unpublished data). It should be noted that PMA and TNFα also enhanced CAT expression in such transfection experiments. Similar results with the HIV κ binding site have recently been reported by (46).

Recently, Baeuerle and Baltimore (47, 48) made the important observation that NF-κB exists in the cytoplasm of unstimulated cells in an inactive form. Using denaturing agents or dissociating agents, these investigators were able to convert to cytosolic inactive form of NF-κB to a form that possesses the ability to bind a DNA fragment containing the κ Ig enhancer sequence. The inactive state of the cytosolic form of NF-κB is the result of its association with a 60-70 kD protein, termed IκB, that binds to NF-κB and masks its DNA-binding activity. In view of our findings on the induction of cAMP and the activation of NF-κB by IL-1, as well as the well-characterized effect of cAMP on the activation of type A protein kinases, we were intrigued by the possibility that cAMP-activated protein kinases might be directly involved in the IL-1-induced activation of NF-κB. We therefore examined the effect of PKA, as well as PKC, on the *in vitro* activation of the precursor form of NF-κB (43). Cytosol from untreated 70Z/3 or YT cells lacks NF-κB binding activity, however, substantial NF-κB binding activity was generated when the cells were treated with PKA for 2-15 min. Identical results were obtained with PKC.

In contrast, PKA and PKC did not activate NF-κB in nuclear extracts from unstimulated cells. Furthermore, when nuclei from unstimulated cells were incubated with PKA- or PKC-treated cytosol for 30 min at 30°C, NF-κB was translocated into the nuclei. This translocation did not occur at 4°C and was inhibited by wheat germ agglutinin (WGA), but not by concanavalin A (con A). The latter finding is most interesting since the transport of a number of nuclear proteins can be blocked by WGA, but not by con A (49-51). In addition, an antibody directed against by acidic amino acid sequence in nuclear pore glycoproteins involved in transport (52) also blocked the nuclear transport of NF-κB. Our findings support the conclusion that NF-κB exists in the cytoplasm of unstimulated 70Z/3 and YT cells in an inactive form that may be converted by exposure to PKA or PKC to an active DNA-binding form that can translocate to the nucleus. These results provide additional support for the hypothesis that the activation of κ Ig and IL-2Rα gene transcription by IL-1 may be mediated via cAMP and the subsequent activation of PKA. Furthermore, these results provide at least one explanation for the overlap in actions between IL-1 and phorbol esters, namely a common event--NF-κB activation and nuclear translocation.

Since NF-κB is not the only DNA binding protein whose activity is regulated by protein kinases, we must consider the possibility that IL-1 may modulate specific gene transcription by regulatory proteins in addition to NF-κB. For example, Kovacs *et al.* (53) demonstrated that IL-1 can induce *c-fos* expression in T lymphocytes. The *c-fos* gene contains a cAMP response element, distinct from the NF-κB binding site, that is involved in the control of *c-fos* gene transcription (54). It is possible that the activation of *c-fos* gene transcription by IL-1 may proceed via a cAMP response element binding protein rather than NF-κB. Furthermore, Cousins and Leinart (55) have demonstrated that IL-1 induces a large increase in metallothionein I and II gene transcription in liver, bone marrow, and thymus. However, these genes lack NF-κB binding sites. Thus if IL-1 has a direct action on metallothionein transcription -- as opposed to inducing an intermediary cytokine--it must exert its effect via a regulatory DNA-binding protein that is distinct from NF-κB.

In addition to an effect on gene transcription, IL-1 may also regulate the processing, transport, or activity of specific precursor or mature mRNA species. For example, McKean (56) reported that IL-1 enhances IL-2 and IL-3 mRNA accumulation in LBRM 33 cells stimulated with mitogen or antibody against the T cell antigen receptor complex. This enhancing effect of IL-1 was not due to an increased rate of transcription, as detected by the nuclear run-on assay, nor to an increased stability of mature mRNA species. Hagiwara *et al.* (57) have obtained data that may indicate that IL-1 can modulate the synthesis of cytokines and surface molecules by more than one mechanism. By itself, IL-1 was able to induce the transcription of mRNA for IL-2Rα, transforming growth factor β, and *c-myc*. In contrast, IL-1 did not affect the transcription of genes for the cytokines IL-2 and IL-3, or the surface antigens Ly-1 and TY 5, but did enhance the transcription of these genes in the presence of a mitogen.

Alternative Second Messengers in the IL-1 Signal-Transduction Pathway

The data obtained in our studies are consistent with the conclusion that the IL-1 receptor is coupled to adenylate cyclase via a novel PT-sensitive G protein in a number of IL-1-responsive cell types (Figure 1). Our findings also indicate that

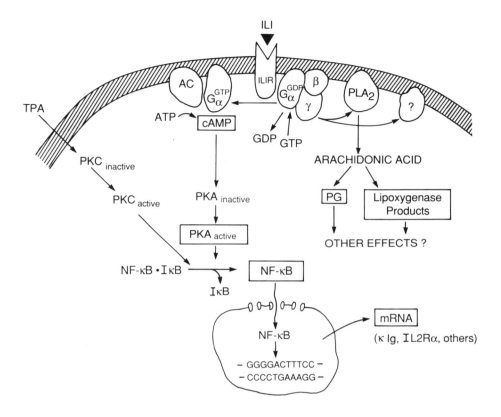

FIG. 1. A model for the IL-1 signal transduction pathway.

IL-1-induced cAMP synthesis may be linked to the activation of specific gene transcriptional events via the activation of the DNA-binding protein, NF-κB. However, we believe that the cAMP-dependent pathway may not be the only operative signal-transduction mechanism for IL-1. We are currently analyzing a variety of IL-1-responsive cell lines for the presence of one or more components of this regulatory pathway. Our preliminary results indicate that IL-1 does not induce cAMP in several T cell lines. However, the IL-1-mediated induction of IL-2 synthesis in these T cell lines is prevented by PT. Thus, it appears that a PT-sensitive G-protein is also involved in the action of IL-1 in these cell lines, but is linked to a second messenger generating system that is distinct from adenylate cyclase.

Although we have made substantial progress in the characterization of at least one signal-transduction pathway for IL-1, it is quite likely that other pathways involving distinct second messengers may be operative in certain cell types. By developing an understanding of the full range of IL-1-induced second messengers, we will be in a much better position to appreciate the overall role of this mediator in immune and inflammatory responses in health and disease.

ACKNOWLEDGMENTS

Portions of this work were supported by Public Health Service grant AI 25836 from the National Institute of Allergy and Infectious Diseases, a gift from RJR-Nabisco, and Public Health Service Oncology Research Center grant CA 12197 from the National Cancer Institute.

REFERENCES

1. Gery, I., Gershon, R. K., and Waksman, B. H. (1972): *J. Exp. Med.* 136:128-142.
2. Deluca, D., and Mizel, S. B. (1986): *J. Immunol.* 137:1435-1441.
3. Mizel, S. B., and Ben-Zvi, A. (1980): *Cell. Immunol.* 54:382-389.
4. Mizel, S. B. (1982): *Immunol. Rev.* 63:51-72.
5. Farrar, W. L., Mizel, S. B., and Farrar, J. J. (1980): *J. Immunol.* 124:1371-1377.
6. Giri, J. G., Kincade, P. W., and Mizel, S. B. (1984): *J. Immunol.* 132:223-228.
7. Stanton, T. H., Maynard, M., and Bomsztyk, K. (1986): *J. Biol. Chem.* 261:5699-5701.
8. Howard, M., and Paul, W. E. (1983): *Ann. Rev. Immunol.* 1:307-333.
9. Mizel, S. B., Dayer, J. M., Krane, S. M., and Mergenhagen, S. E. (1981): *Proc. Natl. Acad. Sci. USA* 138:2474-2477.
10. Schmidt, J. A., Mizel, S. B., Cohen, D., and Green, I. (1982): *J. Immunol.* 128:2177-2182.
11. Rossi, V., Breviario, F., Ghezzi, P., Dejana, E., and Mantovani, A. (1985): *Science* 229:174-176.
12. Dukovich, M., Severin, J. M., White, S. J., Yamazaki, S., and Mizel, S. B. (1986): *Clin. Immunol. Immunopathol.* 38:381-389.
13. Ramadori, G., Sipe, J. D., Dinarello, C. A., Mizel, S. B., and Colten, H. R. (1985): *J. Exp. Med.* 162:930-942.
14. Gowen, M., Wood, D. D., Ihrie, E. J., McGuire, M. K. B., and Russel, G. (1983): *Nature* 306:378-380.
15. Bevilacqua, M. P., Pober, J. S., Majeau, G. R., Cotran, R. S., and Gimbrone, M. A., Jr. (1984): *J. Exp. Med.* 160:618-623.
16. Dinarello, C. A. (1984): *Rev. Infect. Dis.* 6:51-95.
17. Dower, S. K., Call, S. M., Gillis, S., and Urdal, D. L. (1986): *Proc. Natl. Acad. Sci. USA* 83:1060-1064.
18. Dower, S. K., Kronheim, S. R., March, C. J., Conlon, P. J., Hopp, T. P., Gillis, S., and Urdal, D. L. (1985): *J. Exp. Med.* 162:501-515.
19. Kilian, P. L., Kaffka, K. L., Stern, A. S., Woehle, D., Benjamin, W. R., Dechiara, T. M., Gubler, U., Farrar, J. J., Mizel, S. B., and Lomedico, P. T. (1986): *J. Immunol.* 136:4509-4514.
20. Matsushima, K., Akahoshi, T., Yamada, M., Furutani, Y., and Oppenheim, J. J. (1986): *J. Immunol.* 136:4496-4502.
21. Bird, T. S., and Saklatvala, J. (1986): *Nature* 324:263-266.
22. Mizel, S. B., Kilian, P., Lewis, J. C., Paganelli, K. A., and Chizonitte, R. A. (1987): *J. Immunol.* 138:2906-2912.
23. Rhyne, J. A., Mizel, S. B., Taylor, R. G., Chedid, M., and McCall, C. E. (1988): *Clin. Immunol. Immunopathol.* 48:354-361.
24. Abraham, R. T., Ho, S. N., Barna, T. J., and McKean, J. (1987): *J. Biol. Chem.* 25:2719-2728.
25. Avissar, S., Stenzel, K. H., and Novogrodsky, A. (1985): *Cell. Immunol.* 96:462-471.
26. Mukaida, N., Kasahara, T., Yagisawa, H., Shioiri-Nakano, K., and Kawai, T. (1987): *J. Immunol.* 139:3321-3329.
27. Shirakawa, F., Yamashita, U., Chedid, M., and Mizel, S. B. (1988): *Proc. Natl. Acad. Sci. USA* 85:8201-8205.
28. Shirakawa, F., Chedid, M., Suttles, J., Pollok, B. A., and Mizel, S. B. (1989): *Mol. Cell. Biol.* 9:959-964.

29. Shirakawa, F., Tanaka, Y., Eto, S., Suzuki, H., Yodoi, J., and Yamashita, U. (1986): *J. Immunol.* 137:551-556.
30. Chedid, M., Shirakawa, F., Naylor, P., and Mizel, S. B. (1989): *J. Immunol.* 142:4301-4306.
31. Zhang, Y., Lin, J. -X., and Vilcek, J. (1988): *Proc. Natl. Acad. Sci. USA* 85:6802-6805.
32. Lee, J. C., Truneh, A., Smith, M. F., Jr., and Tsang, K. Y. (1987): *J. Immunol.* 139:1935-1938.
33. Gilman, A. G. (1987): *Ann. Rev. Biochem.* 56:615-649.
34. Spiegel, A., Carter, A., Brann, M., Collins, R., Goldsmith, P., Simonds, W., Vinitsky, R., Eide, B., Rossiter, K., Weinstein, L., and Woodard, C. (1988): *Recent Progress in Hormone Research* 44:337-373.
35. Sen, R., and Baltimore, D. (1986): *Cell* 47:921-928.
36. Sen, R., and Baltimore, D. (1986): *Cell* 46:705-716.
37. Queen, C., Foster, J., Stauber, C., and Stafford, J. (1986): *Immunol. Rev.* 89:49-68.
38. Atchison, M. L., and Perry, R. P. (1987): *Cell* 48:121-128.
39. Scheidereit, C., Heguy, A., and Roeder, R. G. (1987): *Cell* 51:783-793.
40. Lenardo, M., Pierce, J. W., and Baltimore, D. (1987): *Science* 236:1573-1577.
41. Nabel, G., and Baltimore, D. (1987): *Nature* 326:711-713.
42. Cross, S. L., Holden, N. F., Lenardo, M. J., and Leonard, W. J. (1989): *Science* 244:466-469.
43. Shirakawa, F., and Mizel, S. B. (1989): *Mol. Cell. Biol.* 9:2424-2430.
44. Hoyos, B., Ballard, D. W., Bohnlein, E., Siekevitz, M., and Green, W. C. (1989): *Science* 244:457-460.
45. Lowenthal, J. W., Bohnlein, E., Ballard, D. W., and Greene, W. C. (1988): *Proc. Natl. Acad. Sci. USA* 85:4468-4472.
46. Osborn, L., Kunkel, S., and Nabel, G. J. (1989): *Proc. Natl. Acad. Sci. USA* 86:2336-2340.
47. Baeuerle, P. A., and Baltimore, D. (1988): *Cell* 53:211-217.
48. Baeuerle, P. A., and Baltimore, D. (1988): *Science* 242:540-546.
49. Finlay, D. R., Newmeyer, D. D., Price, T. M., and Forbes, D. J. (1987): *J. Cell. Biol.* 104:189-200.
50. Yoneda, Y., Imamoto-Sonabe, N., Yamaizumi, M., and Uchida, T. (1987): *Exp. Cell. Res.* 173:586-595.
51. Newmeyer, D. D., and Forbes, D. J. (1988): *Cell* 52:641-653.
52. Yoneda, Y., Imamoto-Sonabe, N., Matsuoka, Y., Iwamoto, R., Kiho, Y., and Uchida, T. (1988): *Science* 242:275-278.
53. Kovacs, E. J., Oppenheim, J. J., and Young, H. A. (1986): *J. Immunol.* 137:3649-3651.
54. Roesler, W. J., Vandenbark, G. R., and Hanson, R. W. (1988): *J. Biol. Chem.* 263:9063-9066.
55. Cousins, R. J., and Leinart, A. S. (1988): *FASEB J.* 2:2884-2890.
56. McKean, D. J., Ho, S. N., and Abraham, R. T. (1989): *FASEB J.* 3:A477.
57. Hagiwara, H., Hang, H. -J. S., Arai, N., Herzemberg, L. A., Arai, K. I., and Zlotnik, A. (1987): *J. Immunol.* 138:2514-2519.

Molecular Aspects of Immune Response and Infectious Diseases, edited by H. Kiyono, E. Jirillo, and C. DeSimone. Raven Press, Ltd., New York, © 1990.

2

Interleukin-4: Production by Mast Cell Lines and by Non-B, Non-T Cells

S. Z. Ben-Sasson*+, G. Le Gros*, M. Plaut‡, D. Conrad§, F. D. Finkelman¶ and W. E. Paul*

Laboratory of Immunology, National Institute of Allergy and Infectious Diseases, National Institutes of Health, Bethesda, MD 20892, USA; the +Lautenberg Center for Tumor Biology, Hebrew University-Hadassah Medical Center, Jerusalem, Israel; the ‡Department of Medicine, Johns Hopkins University School of Medicine, Baltimore, MD 21239; the §Department of Microbiology, Medical College of Virginia, Richmond, VA 23298; and the ¶Department of Medicine, Uniformed Services University of the Health Sciences, Bethesda, MD 20814, USA.

INTRODUCTION

Interleukin-4 is a member of a group of molecules, the lymphokines, that are potent regulators of immune responses and of the growth and differentiation of hematopoietic progenitor cells. Among these molecules, a set can be recognized that are genetically linked and which are often produced by the same cell types. These molecules are interleukin-4 (IL-4), interleukin-5 (IL-5), interleukin-3 (IL-3), and granulocyte-macrophage colony stimulating factor (GM-CSF). The genes for these lymphokines are linked to one another on chromosome 11 in the mouse (1-3) and on the long arm of chromosome 5 in the human (4). For simplicity, these will be referred to as the "IL-4 family of lymphokines." In rodents, T cell lines of the T_{H2} type produce each of the members of the IL-4 family but fail to produce three of the other lymphokines generally regarded as principally of T cell origin, interleukin-2 (IL-2), interferon gamma (IFNγ), and lymphotoxin (LT) (5). In addition, each of the members of the IL-4 family is a potent regulatory of growth and/or differentiation of hematopoietic progenitors. Hematopoietic growth control is usually regarded as the main functions of IL-3 and GM-CSF, but IL-5 is also a potent eosinophil differentiation factor (6) and IL-4 has multiple actions on several hematopoietic lineages (7), including a role as a co-stimulant of mast cell growth (8, 9).

PRODUCTION OF IL-4 BY TRANSFORMED MAST CELL LINES

Although the members of the IL-4 family are usually regarded as mainly, if not exclusively, produced by T lymphocytes, data is now emerging that indicates that the members of the IL-4 family can also be produced by other hematopoietic lineage cells, most notably transformed and non-transformed mast cells. We reported that several transformed mast cell lines expressed mRNA for IL-4 and secreted this molecule (10). Among these were both lines that had been intentionally transformed with Abelson MuLV and spontaneous transformants, including the mast cell line P815. Since IL-4 has activity as a co-stimulant of the growth of factor-dependent mast cell lines *in vitro* (8) and in the formation of mast cell colonies in soft agar (9), one possible explanation for the production of IL-4 by transformed lines was that the lymphokine acted as an autocrine growth factor and its production was thus involved in the transformation process. Although it is difficult to completely exclude this possibility, the finding that monoclonal anti-IL-4 antibody did not inhibit the growth of several of these lines and that excess exogenous IL-4 did not enhance their growth rate strongly suggested that autocrine production of IL-4 was not essential to the transformation process. That led to the consideration that IL-4 production by transformed mast cell lines might reflect the capacity of non-transformed mast cells to produce the lymphokine.

FACTOR-DEPENDENT MAST CELL LINES PRODUCE LYMPHOKINES IN RESPONSE TO CALCIUM IONOPHORES AND Fcε RECEPTOR CROSS-LINKAGE

Some precedent existed for the production of lymphokines by non-lymphoid hematopoietic cells in work of Le Gros *et al.* (11) on production of lymphokines by the factor-dependent myeloid line FDC/1. This IL-3 dependent cell line synthesizes DNA in the absence of exogenous IL-3 upon addition of antigen-antibody complexes. It was shown that FDC/1 cells produced IL-3, IL-4 and GM-CSF in response to stimulation with immune complexes and subsequent work suggests that this stimulation was mediated by cross-linkage of Fcγ receptors (FcγR$_{II}$).

To examine the possibility that non-transformed mast cells could be stimulated to produce IL-4, a series of IL-3 dependent mast cell lines, including CFTL-12, CFTL-15, CFTL-17 and PT-18 were tested. The growth of each of these lines is factor-dependent. All grow in response to IL-3 and IL-4 generally enhances their growth rate; variants of CFTL-12 exist that can grow in IL-4 alone. Treatment of CFTL-12 cells with ionomycin (0.4 μM to 1.0 μM) causes striking DNA synthesis in the absence of exogenous lymphokines (12). This growth response of CFTL-12 is due to autocrine production of IL-3 and IL-4. The evidence supporting this is 1) cyclosporin A, an inhibitor of transcription of several lymphokine genes, blocks DNA synthesis in response to ionomycin but has no effect on the growth of CFTL-12 cells in response to IL-3; 2) supernatant fluids of CFTL-12 cells stimulated with ionomycin contain both IL-3 and IL-4; 3) a combination of monoclonal antibodies to IL-3 and IL-4 inhibit the ionomycin stimulated growth of CFTL-12 cells. These effects are also mediated by another calcium ionophore, A23187 (12).

The capacity of calcium ionophores to cause CFTL-12 cells, as well as CFTL-15, CFTL-17 and PT-18, to produce lymphokines strongly suggested that elevation of cytosolic calcium concentration ([Ca^2]$_i$) could lead to IL-3 and IL-4 production in mast cell lines. Cross-linkage of high affinity Fcε receptors (FcεR$_I$) on mast cells and basophils is known to elevate [Ca^{2+}]$_i$ (13). Since the long term factor-dependent mast cell lines have relatively large numbers of high affinity $Fc\varepsilon R_I$, the capacity of receptor cross-linkage to cause DNA synthesis and lymphokine production by these factor-dependent lines was tested. The cells were sensitized by incubation with a mouse monoclonal IgE anti-dinitrophenyl (DNP) antibody, washed and then exposed to DNP-bovine serum albumin (BSA), containing an average of 23 DNP groups per BSA, or to anti-IgE. These stimulants, which will lead to the release of histamine from CFTL-12 cells, caused the cells to synthesize DNA in the absence of exogenous IL-3. Supernatant fluids from mast cell lines stimulated in this way contained lymphokines. For some of these lines, the concentrations of lymphokines were substantially lower than were found in the supernatants of the same cells stimulated with ionomycin (12).

Although the dose response curves for histamine release and lymphokine production by CFTL-12 cells were generally similar, lymphokine production was not observed for at least one hour after addition of DNP-BSA while histamine production is generally maximal within 15 minutes. Furthermore, steady state levels of mRNA for several lymphokines were strikingly increased in mast cell lines stimulated with ionomycin or by cross-linkage of high affinity $Fc\varepsilon R_I$. This, together with the observation that cyclosporin A strikingly inhibits lymphokine production in response to $Fc\varepsilon R_I$ cross-linkage, strongly argues that lymphokine production depends upon new transcription in response to the cross-linking signal.

MAST CELL LINES PRODUCE A SET OF LYMPHOKINES SIMILAR TO THAT PRODUCED BY T_{H2} CELLS

An analysis of biological activity and mRNA of the four separate mast cell lines indicates that stimulation of sensitized cells by cross-linkage of $Fc\varepsilon R_I$ leads to the production of IL-3, IL-4, IL-5 and GM-CSF. In addition to the production of each of the members of the IL-4 family, stimulated mast cell lines also produce IL-6, IL-1, macrophage inflammatory peptides and $TNF\alpha$ or a related molecule (12, 14, 15).

One of the most interesting features of the production of the members of the IL-4 family of lymphokines by mast cell lines is that these lymphokines have functions that are compatible with their playing important roles in regulating "allergic inflammatory" responses. IL-3 is the major mast cell growth factor (16); IL-4 is required for switching to IgE production both *in vitro* and *in vivo* (17, 18) and also is a co-factor in the growth of mast cells (8, 9); and IL-5 is the major eosinophil differentiation factor (6). Thus, the observation that a series of mast cell lines produce substantial amounts of lymphokines, particularly members of the IL-4 family, raises the possibility that mast cells may be an important regulator of the immunity associated with allergic and anti-parasite responses.

SPLENIC NON-B, NON-T CELLS PRODUCE IL-4 IN RESPONSE TO PLATE-BOUND IgE

In order to gain more insight into the production of lymphokines by mast cells or related cell types, it was necessary to determine whether cells existed in normal mice that had the property of producing these factors in response to cross-linkage of Fcε receptors. It was observed that among the non-B, non-T cells found in the spleen of naive mice, there were cells that produced IL-4 when cultured on dishes to which IgE had been adsorbed. The capacity of such plate-bound (PB)-IgE to elicit IL-4 production from splenic non-B, non-T cells is due to cross-linkage of a high affinity Fcε receptor. Thus, splenic non-B, non-T cells can be sensitized with monoclonal IgE anti-DNP at 1 μg/ml, washed, cultured for two hours at room temperature, and washed again. These cells release IL-4 when cultured with DNP-BSA; the dose response curve for IL-4 production by non-B, non-T cells is similar to that observed for sensitized CFTL-12 cells. These results strongly suggest that cells in the non-B, non-T cell pool bearing high affinity Fcε receptors, presumably $Fc\varepsilon R_I$, are responsible for IL-4 production in response to PB-IgE. Moreover, the response to PB-IgE can be inhibited by soluble IgE; 50% inhibition is achieved with 1 μg/ml. This result is consistent with the receptor being of high affinity and indicates that cross-linkage of the receptor is necessary for the stimulation of IL-4 production by non-B, non-T cells.

IL-3 ENHANCES THE PRODUCTION OF IL-4 BY NON-B, NON-T CELLS

Although splenic non-B, non-T cells from naive animals can produce IL-4 in response to PB-IgE, the amount produced is relatively modest. However, if the cells are cultured with IL-3 and PB-IgE, a striking increase in IL-4 production is observed. Indeed, in the presence of IL-3, the cells produce IL-4 in response to PB-IgG1, PB-IgG2a and PB-IgG2b as well as to PB-IgE. The PB-IgG's appear to stimulate IL-4 production through cross-linkage of an Fc receptor different from that involved in the response to PB-IgE. Stimulation by PB-IgG2a is not inhibited by soluble IgE even at 1 mg/ml but is blocked by 2.4G2, a monoclonal antibody to mouse $Fc\gamma R_{II}$ (19). The effect of IL-3 in enhancing IL-4 production by non-B, non-T cells is quite specific. No effect is seen in response to IL-1, IL-2, IL-5, IL-6, IL-7, or IFNγ. GM-CSF occasionally has a very modest inducing effect.

IL-3 pretreatment of splenic non-B, non-T cells prepares these cells to make an enhanced IL-4 response to stimulation with PB-IgE. This effect occurs even if the cells have been irradiated indicating that the effect of IL-3 is not mediated by expansion of a small subpopulation of cells. Furthermore, IL-3 treatment of mice over a period of three days results in a non-B, non-T cell population that shows enhanced production of IL-4 in response to PB-IgE, even without the presence of additional IL-3.

TREATMENT OF MICE WITH ANTI-IgD ENHANCES IL-4 PRODUCING CAPACITY OF THEIR NON-B, NON-T CELLS

Injection of goat anti-IgD antibodies into mice leads to a striking polyclonal activation of the immune system, presumably due to the binding of anti-IgD to virtually all the B cells, the activation of those cells, the subsequent appearance of T cells specific for goat IgG antigenic determinants, and T cell-B cell interactions potentially involving a large fraction of the B cell population (20). The non-B, non-T cell population in such mice is a larger percentage of the spleen cells than in normal mice and the production of IL-4 from a fixed cell number is often ten- to twenty-fold greater than in naive animals. This together with the fact that the spleens of the animals are much larger than those of naive donors indicates that the IL-4 producing capacity of the non-B, non-T cells in the spleen of an "anti-IgD mouse" may be fifty to one hundred times that of a control non-injected mouse. Not only is there a great increase in the IL-4 producing capacity, non-B, non-T cells from spleens of anti-IgD mice show a greater degree of IL-3 independence in production of IL-4 upon stimulation of PB-Igs.

This IL-3 independent component suggests that the *in vivo* immune response has caused differentiation in at least some non-B, non-T cells so that they are no longer IL-3-dependent, much as *in vitro* or *in vivo* treatment with IL-3 induces such a state. It seems likely that exposure to IL-3 produced by T cells during *in vivo* responses to anti-IgD is responsible for the relative IL-3-independence of these cells, but that has not been directly demonstrated.

Mice injected with anti-IgD display striking T cell-dependent increases in serum IgE levels, often 100-fold or more (21). Treatment of these animals with monoclonal anti-IL-4 antibodies inhibits the IgE increase, indicating that IL-4 plays an important role in the *in vivo* production of IgE (18). The substantial increase in IL-4 producing capacity of non-B, non-T cells in anti-IgD mice may contribute to the induction of serum IgE increases but one must also bear in mind that there is a comparable increase in the IL-4 producing capacity of T cells in these mice.

MICE INFECTED WITH NIPPOSTRONGLYLUS BRASILIENSIS HAVE STRIKING INCREASES IN IL-4 PRODUCING CAPACITY OF NON-B, NON-T CELLS

Infections with nematode parasites often leads to striking increases in serum IgE levels. *Nippostrongylus brasiliensis* (Nb) is widely used as an experimental model infection system. BALB/c mice infected with Nb larvae show striking increases (~300-fold) in serum IgE levels, which are completely blocked by treatment with anti-IL-4 antibody (18). Nb-infected mice show substantial increases in the percentage of spleen cells in the non-B, non-T compartment (up to 25% of spleen cells); marked increases (on a per cell basis) in the IL-4 producing capacity of the non-B, non-T cells (~50-fold) and increased spleen sizes (~2-fold). This indicates that, like anti-IgD mice, Nb-infected animals have a massive increase in IL-4 producing capacity of their splenic non-B, non-T cells (as much as 500-fold).

Non-B, non-T cells from Nb infected animals make substantial amounts of IL-4 in the absence of IL-3. In addition, these cells can be stimulated to secrete IL-4 by anti-IgE antibodies, indicating that the non-B, non-T cells in such animals have Fcε receptors that are occupied by IgE. Furthermore, antigenic extracts prepared from Nb larvae elicit IL-4 production by non-B, non-T cells from Nb-infected mice, suggesting that antigen can cross-link antibodies bound to Fc receptors and can thus stimulate IL-4 production. These striking changes in the non-B, non-T population in infected animals suggest that these cells may have an important role to play in such infections.

LYMPHOKINES PRODUCED BY NON-B, NON-T CELLS

In addition to IL-4, non-B, non-T cells have the capacity to produce IL-3. Cells from naive mice produce small amounts of IL-3 in response to PB-IgE. Cells from "anti-IgD mice" produce considerably more IL-3. The capacity of IL-3 to enhance IL-3 production by non-B, non-T cells has not yet been studied. In addition to IL-3, non-B, non-T cells produce small amounts of IL-5 and GM-CSF in response to PB-IgE. However, these cells fail to produce IL-2 or IFNγ. Thus, splenic non-B, non-T cells from anti-IgD-treated mice have a pattern of lymphokine production similar to factor-dependent long term murine mast cells lines and to T_{H2} type helper T cell lines.

CHARACTERIZATION OF IL-4-PRODUCING NON-B, NON-T CELLS

IL-4 production can be elicited in non-B, non-T cell populations obtained from spleen and bone marrow of normal mice as well as from anti-IgD mice and Nb mice. In naive, immunized or infected animals, lymph node, thymus and peritoneal cavity preparations of non-B, non-T cells fail to produce IL-4 in response to PB-Igs in the presence or absence of IL-3. However, non-B, non-T cells prepared from lungs of Nb-infected mice do show substantial capacity to produce IL-4.

Depletion of Mac-1-bearing cells from the non-B, non-T cells population does not diminish the IL-4-producing capacity of the residual cells. Similarly, removal of cells bearing asialo-GM1 (aGM1), which removes cells with NK activity, tends to enhance IL-4 producing capacity. Separation of non-B, non-T cells on Percoll density gradients reveals that virtually all the IL-4-producing capacity is found in cells that band between 50 and 60% Percoll (i.e., intermediate density cells). Cells in this population are relatively large with considerable basophilic cytoplasm. The phenotypic analysis of these cells, to this time, indicates that a population that is CD3-, CD4-, CD8-, Thy 1-, B220-. Ia-, Mac 1- and aGM1- can produce IL-4 in response to PB-IgE.

The capacity of non-B, non-T cells to retain IgE with which they have been sensitized upon culture at 37°C for several hours and the capacity of low concentrations of soluble IgE to block stimulation by PB-IgE is indicative that the responding cells have a high affinity Fcε receptor. The only receptor known with these properties is FcεR$_I$. Nonetheless, when sensitized cells are stained with fluoresceinated anti-IgE, no positive cells are detected by flow cytometric analysis. This is in keeping with the absence of mature mast cells from the spleen and from the splenic non-B, non-T cell population. One possible explanation is that the cells that produce IL-4 in response to PB-IgE have small numbers of FcεR$_I$ molecules on their membrane, sufficient for stimulation of IL-4 production but too few for detection by a fluorescence cytometric analysis. In turn, since the spleen and the bone marrow are known to contain mast cell precursors (22) and FcεR$_I$ may well be limited in expression to the mast cell and basophil lineages, it is reasonable to propose that the non-B, non-T cells that produce IL-4 in response to PB-IgE are mast cell precursors. Whether the same cells respond to PB-IgG and PB-IgE is not known. However, the original findings of Le Gros *et al.* (11) that the myeloid lineage cell line FDC/1 produced lymphokines upon stimulation with immune complexes raises the possibility that at least some of the IL-4 production in non-B, non-T cell populations stimulated with PB-IgGs comes from myeloid lineage cells.

POTENTIAL SIGNIFICANCE OF IL-4 PRODUCTION BY NON-B, NON-T CELLS

The experimental results reviewed here demonstrate that long term mast cell lines and a population of non-B, non-T cells in the spleen and bone marrow of normal and immune mice produce IL-4 in response to cross-linkage of a high affinity Fcε receptor or of an Fcγ receptor. Infection with Nb or injection of anti-

IgD antibodies, two treatments known to cause massive elevation in serum IgE concentrations, cause striking increases in the IL-4-producing capacity of non-B, non-T cells as well as leading to the appearance of a substantial capacity to produce IL-4 without the addition of IL-3. This is consistent with the IL-4-producing non-B, non-T cells playing some role in the immune responses associated with IgE elevation and with helminthic infection. Although it would be premature to specify such a role, it is striking to recall that T cell IL-4 production is stimulated by a membrane-bound ligand (antigen-derived peptide bound to a class II or class I major histocompatibility complex molecule). Furthermore, there is evidence that IL-4 production in response to activation of T cells may be focused upon the antigen-presenting cell. By contrast, non-B, non-T cells use an antibody as their receptor for antigen. Thus, they could recognize a soluble ligand and secrete IL-4 and other lymphokines into the extracellular fluid and may produce these lymphokines for action at a distance rather than as exclusive autocrine or paracrine factors.

In addition, the receptors of IL-4-producing non-B, non-T cells are non-clonally distributed. Thus, either through the binding of immune complexes to Fc receptors or of multivalent antigens to antibodies already bound to Fc receptors, non-B, non-T cells may markedly amplify T cell lymphokine production by bringing many additional cells into play. This might indicate that T cells become activated as a result of interacting with antigen and antigen-presenting cells. Such activated T cells not only mediate direct helper functions but may also recruit non-B, non-T cells capable of producing IL-4 through the production by the T cell of IL-3. This event could result in a strong amplification of a T cell dependent immune response that is characterized by the production of the IL-4 family of lymphokines.

A final point that should be considered is that non-B, non-T cells can respond to immune complexes. Consequently, they may be an important source of lymphokine production at the site of immune complex deposition and thus may strikingly contribute to local inflammatory responses in such circumstances. This may be particularly important in systemic autoimmune diseases in which T cell production of IL-3 might keep the non-B, non-T cells in a state competent to produce IL-4.

Furthermore, as noted above, non-B, non-T cells from anti-IgD mice produce IL-3 as well as IL-4 in response to cross-linkage of Fcε receptors. Thus, once activated, the non-B, non-T cells may be able to sustain themselves in a state competent to produce IL-4 without the need for an exogenous source of IL-3. Clearly, the potential importance of non-B, non-T cells in lymphokine production in autoimmune diseases requires a detailed examination of the number and properties of these cells in such mice.

SUMMARY

Interleukin-4 and a set of related lymphokines (IL-5, IL-3 and GM-CSF) are not only produced by activated T cells but can also be secreted by long term mast cell lines. The latter secrete lymphokines in response to stimulation with calcium ionophores or to cross-linkage of high affinity Fcε receptors, presumably $FcεR_I$. In spleens and bone marrow of normal mice, a population of non-B, non-T lymphocytes exist that have the capacity to produce both IL-4 and IL-3 in response to IgE that has been adsorbed to a surface. Their production of IL-4 is markedly enhanced by treatment with IL-3 and cells that have been treated with IL-3 also produce IL-4 in response to surface adsorbed IgG1, IgG2a and IgG2b. Mice that have been injected with anti-IgD antibodies or infected with *Nippostrongylus brasiliensis* larvae display a striking increase in the capacity of their non-B, non-T cells to produce of IL-4 and IL-3 in response to PB-IgE and IgGs. Furthermore, their non-B, non-T cells produce substantial amounts of IL-4 in response to PB-IgE or PB-IgG even in the absence of IL-3. The production of IL-4 and other members of the IL-4 family of lymphokines by mast cells and by non-B, non-T cells may have importance both in allergic and anti-parasite responses as well as in local inflammatory responses to immune complexes.

REFERENCES

1. Barlow, D. P., Bucan, M., Lehrach, H., Hogan, B. L. M., and Gough, N. M. (1987): *EMBO J.* 6:617-623.
2. D'Eustachio, P., Brown, M., Watson, C., and Paul, W. E. (1988): *J. Immunol.* 141:3067-3071.
3. Lee, J. S., Campbell, H. D., Kozak, C. A., and Young, I. G. (1989): *Somat. Cell. Mol. Genet.* 15:143-152.
4. van Leeuwen, B. H., Martinson, M. E., Webb, G. C., and Young, I. G. (1989): *Blood* 73:1142-1148.
5. Mosmann, T. R., Cherwinski, H., Bond, M. W., Giedlin, M. A., and Coffman, R. L. (1986): *J. Immunol.* 136:2348-2357.
6. Sanderson, C. J., O'Garra, A., Warren, D. J., and Klaus, G. G. (1986): *Proc. Natl. Acad. Sci.* 83:437-440.
7. Peschel, C., Paul, W. E., Ohara, J., and Green, I. (1987): *Blood* 70:254-263.
8. Mosmann, T. R., Bond, M. W., Coffman, R. L., Ohara, J., and Paul, W. E. (1986): *Proc. Natl. Acad. Sci.* 83:5654-5658.
9. Hamaguchi, Y., Kanakura, Y., Fujita, J., Takeda, S. -I., Nakano, T., Tarui, S., Honjo, T., and Kitamura, Y. (1987): *J. Exp. Med.* 165:268-281.
10. Brown, M. A., Pierce, J. A., Watson, C. J., Falco, J., Ihle, J. N., and Paul, W. E. (1987): *Cell* 50:809-818.
11. Le Gros, G., Le Gros, J., and Watson, J. D. (1987): *J. Immunol.* 134:422-428.
12. Plaut, M., Pierce, J. H., Watson, C. J., Hanley-Hyde, J., Nordan, R. P., and Paul, W. E. (1989): *Nature* 339:64-67.
13. Metzger, H., Alcaraz, G., Hohman, R., Kinet, J. -P., Pribulda, V., and Quarto, R. (1986): *Ann. Rev. Immunol.* 4:419-470.
14. Wodnar-Fillipowicz, A., Heusser, C. H., and Maroni, C. (1986): *Nature* 339:150-152.
15. Burd, P. R., Rogers, H. W., Gordon, J. R., Martin, C. A., Jayaraman, S., Wilson, S. D., Dvorak, A. M., Galli, S. J., and Dorf, M. E. (1986): *J. Exp. Med.* 170:245-257.
16. Ihle, J. N., Keller, J., Oroszlan, S., Henderson, L. E., Copeland, T. D., Fitch, F., Prystowsky, M. B., Goldwasser, E., Schrader, J. W., Palaszynski, E., Dy, M., and Lebel, B. (1983): *J. Immunol.* 131:282-287.
17. Coffman, R. L., Ohara, J., Bond, M. W., Carty, J., Zlotnik, A., and Paul, W. E. (1986): *J. Immunol.* 136:4538-4541.
18. Finkelman, F. D., Kotana, I., Urban, J., Snapper, C., Ohara, J., and Paul, W. E. (1986): *Proc. Natl. Acad. Sci.* 83:9674-9678.
19. Unkeless, J. (1979): *J. Exp. Med.* 150:580-596.
20. Finkelman, F. D., Scher, I., Mond, J. J., Kessler, S., Kung, J. P., and Metcalf, E. S. (1982): *J. Immunol.* 129:638-646.
21. Finkelman, F. D., Snapper, C. M., Mountz, J. D., and Katona, I. M. (1987): *J. Immunol.* 138:2826-2834.
22. Sakoda, H., and Miro, K. J. (1989): *Exp. Hematol.* 17:791-794.

Molecular Aspects of Immune Response and Infectious Diseases, edited by H. Kiyono, E. Jirillo, and C. DeSimone. Raven Press, Ltd., New York, © 1990.

3

The Immunobiology of Interleukin 6 (IL-6) and Its Receptor

T. Kishimoto, T. Hirano, T. Taga, T. Matsuda, S. Suematsu, M. Hibi, K. Yamasaki, K. Yasukawa and Y. Hirata

Institute for Molecular and Cellular Biology, Osaka University, Suita, Osaka, Japan

IL-6 is a multifunctional cytokine produced by both lymphoid and nonlymphoid cells (1). It was originally identified as a T cell-derived lymphokine that caused the terminal differentiation of activated B cells to antibody producing cells. Molecular cloning of the cDNA (2) and the studies with recombinant molecules demonstrated that IL-6 has a wide variety of biological functions and that its target cells are not restricted to normal B cells. Responses are also seen in T cells (3), plasmacytomas (4), hepatocytes (5), hematopoietic stem cells (6), megakaryocytes (7) and nerve cells (8) (Figure 1).

Of particular interest is that IL-6 is a potent growth factor for murine plasmacytomas. This observation suggests to us that constitutive expression of IL-6 or its receptor could be responsible for the generation of human multiple myelomas. The studies with recombinant IL-6 and anti-IL-6 antibody demonstrated that i) IL-6 augments *in vitro* growth of myeloma cells freshly isolated from patients, ii) all myeloma cells produce IL-6 and express IL-6 receptors and iii) anti-IL-6 inhibits the *in vitro* growth of myeloma cells. This is a direct evidence that an autocrine loop is operating in oncogenesis of human myelomas (9). The involvement of IL-6 in the generation of myelomas was further confirmed in transgenic mice with the Eμ-IL-6 gene (10). The constitutive expression of IL-6 in B lineage cells of Eμ-IL-6 transgenic mice induced plasmacytosis.

As expected from its multiple function, IL-6 receptor (IL-6R) is expressed on various tissues and cells but the number of the receptor is extremely low (11). The cDNA for IL-6R was cloned and the deduced amino acid sequence showed that IL-6R consisted of 468 amino acids and the first domain following a signal sequence belonged to the immunoglobulin supergene family (12) (Figure 2). The rest of the extracellular portion was shown to be a member of the cytokine receptor family to

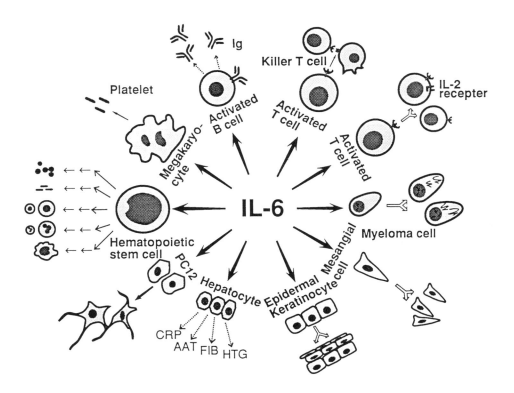

FIG. 1. Multifunction of IL-6.

which IL-2Rβ (13), IL-4R (14), EpoR (15) and GM-CSFR (16) belong (Figure 2). Intracytoplasmic portion of the IL-6R with 82 amino acids did not have any unique structures for signal transduction, such as tyrosine kinase domain, although IL-6 functions as a potent growth factor for plasmacytoma / myeloma. This finding suggests an existence of a signal transducing molecule associating with the receptor. A monoclonal antibody against IL-6R could precipitate a single polypeptide chain with a Mr of 80k which was involved in binding with IL-6. However, incubation of cells with IL-6 at 37°C could induce the association of IL-6R and a second polypeptide chain with a Mr of 130 k (gp130), which did not have ligand-binding activity (17). Human IL-6R could associate with the murine gp130 homolog and was functional in murine cells. Mutant IL-6R lacking intracytoplasmic portion could associate with gp130 and transduce the signal. The results indicate that the association between IL-6R and gp130 is responsible for signal transduction. This was further confirmed with recombinant soluble IL-6R. A soluble IL-6R lacking transmembrane and intracytoplasmic domains could interact with gp130 in the presence of IL-6 and mediate IL-6 signals. Interaction

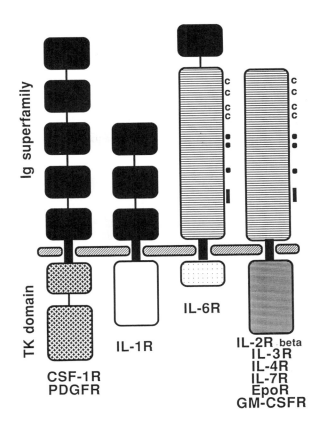

FIG. 2. Structural relationship between cytokine receptors. Closed square, immunoglobulin like domain; c and dots, conserved cystein and other amino acid residues in the cytokine receptor family; vertical bar, Tryptophan-Serine-X-Tryptophan-Serine motif in the family.

between a ligand-binding chain and a non-ligand binding but signal transducing chain is an unique mechanism and may be applied for other cytokine systems.

REFERENCES

1. Kishimoto, T. (1989): *Blood* 74:1-10.
2. Hirano, T., Yasukawa, K., Harada, H., Taga, T., Watanabe, Y., Matsuda, T., Kashiwamura, S., Nakajima, K., Koyama, K., Iwamatu, A., Tsunasawa, S., Sakiyama, F., Matsui, H., Takahara, Y., Taniguchi, T., and Kishimoto, T. (1986): *Nature* 324:73-76.
3. Okada, M., Kitahara, M., Kishimoto, S., Matsuda, T., Hirano, T., and Kishimoto, T. (1988): *J. Immunol.* 141:1543-1549.
4. Van Damme, J., Opdenakker, G., Simpson, R. J., Rubira, M. R., Cayphas, S., Vink, A., Billiau, A., and Snick, J. V. (1987): *J. Exp. Med.* 165:914-919.

5.   Andus, T., Geiger, T., Hirano, T., Northoff, H., Ganter, U., Bauer, J., Kishimoto, T., and Heinrich, P. C. (1987): *FEBS Lett.* 221:18-22.
6.   Ikebuchi, K., Wong, G. G., Clark., S. C., Ihle, J. N., Hirai, Y., and Ogawa, M. (1987): *Proc. Natl. Acad. Sci. (USA)* 84:9035-9039.
7.   Ishibashi, T., Kimura, H., Uchida, T., Kariyone, S., Friese, P., and Burstein, S. A. (1989): *Proc. Natl. Acad. Sci. (USA)* 86:5953-5947.
8.   Satoh, T., Nakamura, S., Taga, T., Matsuda, T., Hirano, T., Kishimoto, T., and Kaziro, Y. (1988): *Mol. Cell. Biol.* 8:3546-3549.
9.   Kawano, M., Hirano, T., Matsuda, T., Taga, T., Horii, Y., Iwato, K., Asaoku, H., Tang, B., Tanabe, O., Tanaka, H., Kuramoto, A., and Kishimoto, T. (1988): *Nature* 332:83-87.
10. Suematsu, S., Matsuda, T., Aozasa, K., Akira, S., Nakano, N., Ohno, S., Miyazaki, J., Yamamura, K., Hirano, T., and Kishimoto, T. (1989): *Proc. Natl. Acad. Sci. (USA)* 86:7547-7551.
11. Taga, T., Kawanishi, K., Hardy, R. R., Hirano, T., and Kishimoto, T. (1987): *J. Exp. Med.* 166:967-981.
12. Yamasaki, K., Taga, T., Hirata, Y., Yawata, H., Kawanishi, Y., Seed, B., Taniguchi, T., Hirano, T., and Kishimoto, T. (1988): *Science* 241:825-828.
13. Hatakeyama, M., Tsudo, M., Minamoto, S., Kono, T., Doi, T., Miyata, T., Miyasaka, M., and Taniguchi, T. (1989): *Science* 244:551-556.
14. Mosley, B., Beckmann, M. P., March, C. J., Idzerda, R. L., Gimpel, S. D., VandenBos, T., Friend, D., Alpert, A., Anderson, D., Jackson, J., Wignall, J. M., Smith, C., Gallis, B., Sims, J. E., Urdal, D., Widmer, M. B., Cosman, D., and Park, L. S. (1989): *Cell* 59:335-348.
15. D'Andrea, A., Lodish, H. F., and Wong, G. G. (1989): *Cell* 57:277-285.
16. Gearing, D. P., King, J. A., Gough, N. M., and Nicola, N. A. (1989): *EMBO J.* 8:3677-3684.
17. Taga, T., Hibi, M., Hirata, Y., Yamasaki, K., Yasukawa, K., Matsuda, T., Hirano, T., and Kishimoto, T. (1989): *Cell* 58:573-581.

Molecular Aspects of Immune Response and Infectious Diseases, edited by H. Kiyono, E. Jirillo, and C. DeSimone. Raven Press, Ltd., New York, © 1990.

4

Molecular Characterization of Cytokines and Their Receptors

J. E. Sims

Immunex Corporation, 51 University Street, Seattle, Washington 98101, USA

CHARACTERIZATION OF IL-7

Interleukin 7 (IL-7) was discovered several years ago by Namen *et al.* (1), who was trying to study the differentiation and maturation of B cell precursors using long-term bone marrow cultures of the Whitlock-Witte type. These cultures consist of two types of cells, an adherent stromal layer attached to the tissue culture plastic, which allows the growth of other cells in suspension consisting primarily although not exclusively of immature B cells. In order to study this in more detail, Namen *et al.* wanted to derive a stromal cell line. Namen and Overell were able to do this by transforming one of these stromal cultures with SV40. The cells of this line, called A6, have a typical fibroblast-like appearance and support the growth of small round lymphoid cells that appear to grow on top of the stromal cell layer. Namen found that the stromal cells themselves were not necessary, and that conditioned medium from the stromal cell line was capable of supporting the long-term survival and proliferation of the B cell precursors. In fact, he was able to derive a pre-B cell line that grew in tissue culture over an extended period of time in response to a factor secreted by the stromal cell line.

We were interested in cloning this factor in order to understand it better. Because it was produced in miniscule quantities, the cloning method that we chose was direct expression in mammalian cells. David Cosman at Immunex has generated a series of expression vectors designed to express cDNA molecules at very high levels when transfected into mammalian cells. The high levels of expression are due to the presence of the adenovirus major later promoter and the adenovirus tripartite leader which drive a high level of transcription and translation from the inserted cDNA molecule. The overall scheme for direct expression cloning of IL-7 involved generating a cDNA library from the A6 cell line in a direct expression plasmid, and plating out that cDNA library in relatively small pools of roughly 1000 colonies per plate. DNA made from each of those pools was used to transfect COS cells and, after a three day period to allow for expression of the cDNA clones, the supernatant from these cells was assayed for the ability to support the growth of the pre-B cell line. After a long period of tedious searching, Tony Namen, Ray Goodwin and Steve Lupton found a positive pool (2). The A6 cell line makes about 20 units per ml of IL-7. COS cells transfected with the expression vector alone don't make any, and when they finally found a positive pool, it made a barely detectable level of IL-7, about 5.5 units per ml. After they went back to this pool and broke it down into smaller pools, they found to their satisfaction a considerable enrichment in the level of activity, until a pure cDNA clone was isolated which made approximately 11,000 units per ml of IL-7.

The recombinant IL-7 made in COS cells behaves identically to the natural material made by the A6 cell line, in that it supports the survival and proliferation of B cell precursors over a long period of time in culture. IL-7 supports the survival of classic pre-B cells which have rearranged and are expressing their heavy chains but have not yet rearranged their light chains. In addition, it supports the proliferation of cells at what is presumably an even earlier stage in the B cell lineage, namely those which are B220 positive but have not yet rearranged either of their immunoglobulin genes. However, it does not lead to the proliferation of more mature B cells once they have reached the stage of being surface Ig^+.

When the IL-7 insert was used as a probe to look for mRNA expression in various mouse tissues it was found that message was present not only in spleen and in bone marrow, which is where one would expect to find it, but also in thymus. This raised the question of whether IL-7 supports the growth of T cell precursors as well as B cell precursors, and indeed it does. IL-7 in fact supports the growth of early T cells from either adult thymus or fetal thymus (3, 4). The thymocytes proliferating in response to IL-7 are very early thymocytes, so called double negatives, which express CD3 on the cell surface but do not express CD4 or CD8. IL-7 acts to drive the proliferation of these cells but, as is the case with B cell precursors, it doesn't seem to stimulate their differentiation to a stage at which they express CD4 or CD8. It also seems to be acting directly on these cells rather than inducing some other immediate proliferative factor in that there is no change in expression of interleukin 2 (IL-2) or interleukin 4 (IL-4) genes in these thymocytes, nor do antibodies to IL-2 or IL-4 have any inhibitory effect on proliferation.

IL-7 also seems to act on more mature T cells, unlike the case with B cells. It is a potent proliferative signal for the growth of peripheral blood T cells and splenic T cells although in this instance it usually requires the presence of a co-mitogen, either Con A or PHA, in order to do so, and it seems to be acting through the secretion of IL-2 and the expression of IL-2 receptors on the surface of these cells (5).

INTERACTION OF IL-1 AND IL-1R

If one is interested in knowing how lymphokines influence hematopoiesis or mediate immune or inflammatory responses, it is critical to study not only the ligand but also the ligand binding moiety in order to get a complete understanding of these processes. Interleukin 1 (IL-1) has multiple actions on many different organ systems and cell types. Its primary role seems to be in host defense mechanisms, modulating the immune response, mediating inflammatory reactions and regulating the very early stages of hematopoiesis. A partial list of various cell types that express IL-1 receptors includes cells of the lymphoid and myeloid systems, fibroblasts, skin cells, endothelial cells, and hepatocytes. It is striking that not only is the range of IL-1 responsive cell types very broad, but also that most of these cells express very few IL-1 receptors (IL-1R). With the exception of keratinocytes, under somewhat unusual circumstances, fibroblasts (with typically a few thousand receptors per cell) are by far the most abundant source of IL-1 receptor. More typically there are tens to hundreds of IL-1 receptors per cell, emphasizing the sensitivity of signaling that is mediated by IL-1.

Binding of IL-1α and IL-1β to IL-1R

The first series of experiments were done several years ago by Steve Dower and Dave Urdal at Immunex, although similar experiments have been carried out in a number of laboratories with similar results. These experiments sought to characterize the receptor for IL-1 in its normal conformation in the membranes of the intact cells. Standard radioreceptor assays, in which cells (in this case, EL 4 murine T lymphoma cells) are incubated with increasing amounts of radioactive IL-1, show increasing amounts of IL-1 bound, until the receptors on the cell are saturated. The data can be plotted in the Scatchard coordinate system and give a straight line, which tells that there is a single class if IL-1 binding sites on the EL 4 cells (as is true for most cells expressing IL-1R). The affinity of the IL-1R can be determined from the slope of the line and is about 3×10^9 M^{-1} (6). If one is more used to thinking in terms of dissociation constants, that's about 200 pM, which is quite high affinity.

The next experiments examined the ability of IL-1α and IL-1β to compete for each others' binding (7). Cells are incubated with radioactive IL-1α and increasing amounts of unlabeled IL-1, either α or β. At sufficient concentration, both forms are able to inhibit completely the binding of radioactive IL-1α. The reciprocal experiment done with radioactive IL-1β gives the same answer. One might recall that the two forms of IL-1 are quite dissimilar at the primary structure level. They share only 26% amino acid identity (8) and yet they apparently bind with very similar affinities to the same cell surface receptor molecule.

Physical Characterization and Cloning of IL-1R

Preliminary physical characterization of the receptor molecule was done by crosslinking (6). Cells are incubated with radioactive IL-1, a chemical crosslinker is added to covalently couple the IL-1 to its receptor and the whole complex is run out on an SDS gel. Predominantly one sees a single band that migrates at about 100 kd. If one subtracts the size of the radioactive IL-1 which is about 18 kd, it gives a size for the receptor of about 80 to 82 kd.

We were interested in cloning this receptor in order to characterize it further. Again, because it was expressed at a very low level, it was a very difficult task to purify enough of it to get any protein sequence and it had proved impossible to raise antibodies to it. So once again we have used expression cloning. A cDNA library was made from a relatively rich source of IL-1 receptor, namely the EL 4 cell line, and ligated into a mammalian expression vector. Pools of cDNA clones were transfected with COS cells, and we screened for IL-1 receptor clones by looking for transfected COS cells which could bind greatly increased amounts of radioactive IL-1. Because the COS cells themselves express a low level of IL-1 receptors, about 500 receptors per cell, they give a certain background of bound IL-1. In order to gain greater sensitivity over this background, instead of simply counting the transfected cells in a gamma counter after they had bound radioactive IL-1, we elected to do audioradiography on cell monolayers by incubating the cells with IL-1α and then just putting the whole plate on film. Plates which have been transfected with vector alone, or with a negative pool of cDNA clones, show a uniform grey background due to the binding of IL-1 by the COS cells. When we finally found a positive pool, there were about 25 discrete dark spots on top of the background, which represented individual cells transfected with an IL-1R plasmid expressing high levels of IL-1R on the COS cell surface and which were therefore now binding greatly increased amounts of IL-1. We purified the clone responsible for that phenotype by standard sib selection techniques, until we isolated a single cDNA clone (9). Control experiments showed that the binding induced by that clone is specific, in that it is completely competed by unlabeled IL-1α or unlabeled IL-1β. This shows that we haven't simply cloned something which makes the cells generally sticky.

We sequenced the insert from the cDNA clone and found that it encoded a relatively long reading open frame. While we were cloning the receptor by expression, Carl March at Immunex had succeeded in purifying a small quantity of the natural IL-1R protein from the EL 4 cells and getting an N-terminal amino acid sequence from it of 26 amino acids. This exact same predicted amino acid sequence was found near the N-terminus of the open reading frame of the cDNA clone, confirming that this was indeed a clone for the IL-1R molecule. The insert from this cDNA clone, when hybridized to RNA from EL 4 cells on a Northern blot, gives a single band of about 5 kb. Hybridization to RNA from a variant EL 4 cell line that expresses no IL-1R on its surface shows no RNA present that corresponds to this clone. Similarly, hybridization to RNA from two different fibroblast cell lines that differ by about ten fold in their level of surface IL-1R expression also shows a corresponding variation in mRNA level. That the level of hybridizing RNA correlates with the level of cell surface IL-1R expression, further confirms the identity of the clone.

The predicted amino acid sequence of the open reading frame shows a short signal peptide (to the 5' side of the mature N-terminus of the protein, as determined by direct sequencing) and a single membrane spanning region that separates the molecule into two roughly equal halves. There is an N-terminal half of 319 amino acids that is the extracellular ligand binding part of the molecule and which contains all of the potential sites of N-linked glycosylation, and a C-terminal portion of 217 amino acids which presumably is the cytoplasmic part of the IL-1R and is responsible for mediating signal transduction.

Analysis of Extracellular Domain of Cloned IL-1R

Most of the rest of this article will focus first on the extracellular part of the molecule and then turn to the cytoplasmic portion of the molecule. The ligand binding properties of the recombinant receptor were first studied using transient transfection in COS cells, and compared with the properties of the natural receptor in EL 4 cells. Binding curves and Scatchard plots for the recombinant and the natural IL-1R both give single straight lines and are essentially parallel, showing that the two have indistinguishable affinities. A competition experiment similar to the one described earlier demonstrates that the recombinant as well as the natural receptor binds both IL-1α and IL-1β. Finally, in a surface labeling experiment, the recombinant IL-1 receptor expressed in transfected COS cells is identical in size to the IL-1R in its natural form in EL 4 cells. By these assays, the recombinant receptor and the natural receptor are indistinguishable.

We have gone on to generate a truncated form of the IL-1R that we call a soluble version by introducing a translational stop codon immediately prior to the transmembrane region (10). This produces a molecule which is secreted into the medium rather than being membrane bound. It is stable and soluble in the tissue culture medium and can be purified by affinity chromatography on IL-1 coupled to sepharose. On SDS gels the purified material shows two closely-spaced bands, which is a consequence of slight C-terminal degradation.

We can assay for the soluble receptor by a simple plate binding assay. Tissue culture plates are coated with an antibody to the receptor (using one that doesn't block IL-1 binding) and then incubated with medium containing the soluble IL-1R. The soluble receptor will bind to the antibody, and it can be detected in turn by its ability to bind radioactive IL-1. We can use this plate-binding assay to do the same sort of standard kinetic assays with the soluble receptor molecule as with the full-length receptor, and we get exactly the same answers, namely, that it binds both IL-1α and IL-1β with affinities which are indistinguishable from cell-bound receptor. Thus we can conclude quite conclusively that there is no molecule that is responsible for contributing any of the energy of IL-1 binding other than this soluble, ligand binding part of the cloned receptor.

Examination of the sequence of the IL-1R reveals that the extracellular portion is comprised almost entirely of three immunoglobulin-like domains. In this regard, immunoglobulin domains are composed primarily of two β-sheets held together by a disulfide band. Immunoglobulin molecules and immunoglobulin-like domains interact with other molecules in one of two standard fashions. One way is by means of the loops at the N-terminal end of the domains, which is where in antibody molecules and in T cell receptor molecules the hypervariable regions are located that are responsible for interacting with antigen. It is also the region that is used by the CD2 molecule to interact with its ligand the LFA3 antigen. On the other hand, interactions between immunoglobulin-like domains within immunoglobulin molecules and T cell receptors, or for that matter between MHC class I antigens and β2 microglobulin, are mediated by the β-sheets that form the faces of the Ig domains.

The crystal structure for IL-1β shows a rather symmetrical molecule, a pyramid or or tetrahedron composed primarily of smooth faces of β-sheet (11). While it is pure speculation at the moment, it is tempting to wonder if each of the three Ig domains of the IL-1R can use one of its β-sheets to interact with the β-sheets that form the faces of the IL-1 molecule. We have no real information on this at the moment. However, as a preliminary step toward understanding the interaction between IL-1 and its receptor, we have made precise deletions of each of the three Ig-like domains of the receptor. Those constructs have been transfected into COS cells and their ability to bind radioactive IL-1 ascertained. Deletion of any of the three domains completely abolishes the ability of the receptor to bind either IL-1α or IL-1β (12). We are currently performing saturation mutagenesis on the receptor to define more precisely which amino acids are actually involved in ligand binding.

Biological Characterization of Extracellular Domain of Cloned IL-1R

We have also begun to do biological experiments using the soluble IL-1R construct (13). One of the experimental systems involves injecting a BALB/c mouse in one hind footpad with irradiated allogenic (C57B1/6) spleen cells and, as a control, injecting the other hind footpad with irradiated syngeneic BALB/c spleen cells. After seven days, the draining lymph node in the popliteal fossa is removed. Typically a lymph node in this position weighs about 1 mg. In this sort of response to allogeneic cells, it increases to somewhere between 2 and 4 mg after seven days. The increase in weight reflects an increase in cell number as the immune system responds to the challenge with foreign cells. The lymph node draining the footpad injected with syngeneic cells usually does not change in size.

The increase in lymph node size in the leg injected with allogenic cells can be completely blocked by systemic injection of a sufficient quantity of soluble IL-1R. The soluble receptor can be given intravenously, intraperitoneally or subcutaneously. It is most effective if given on the day prior to injection of the foreign cells, somewhat effective if given on the day of injection, and ineffective on the day following injection. Finally, to prove that the soluble receptor is indeed acting by soaking up endogenously produced IL-1 which is mediating the enlargement of the lymph node, it was shown that the effect can be overcome by co-injecting it with an excess of IL-1. We don't know the mechanism by which IL-1 leads to the enlargement of this lymph node when challenged with foreign cells, but it is clear that injecting the soluble receptor molecule can interfere with the effect of the IL-1 that is endogenously produced and mediating this response, and we might hope that this potentially could be used in chronic inflammatory disease processes such as, perhaps, arthritis.

Characterization of Cytoplasmic Domain of Cloned IL-1R

In this section, we describe the cytoplasmic part of the IL-1R. Thus, we have initially determined the relevance of the molecule that we had cloned. In particular, we wanted to ask whether this molecule is functional in signal transduction. In order to do that we derived stably transformed CHO cell lines that express about 80,000 recombinant IL-1R per cell (14). This is in contrast to the parental CHO cells (or several control transfectants that we made) which express approximately 50 IL-1R per cell. We measured the biological responses of these cells to IL-1 by looking for either production of prostaglandin E2 (PGE_2) or the secretion of granulocyte colony stimulating factor (G-CSF).

The result we got was that the cells which had been transfected with the recombinant IL-1R and were expressing about 1000-fold more IL-1R per cell than the parental CHO cells, were also approximately 1000 times more sensitive to the effects of IL-1 than the parental cells. For example, the control CHO cells require concentrations of about 10^{-10} M IL-1 before they begin to secrete G-CSF, whereas the cells expressing the recombinant receptor respond at about 10^{-13} M IL-1. Similar results were obtained when we examined PGE_2 production. Cells expressing high levels of recombinant IL-1R made PGE_2 in response to 10^{-14} M IL-1, whereas the parental CHO cells failed to respond at IL-1 concentrations of less than 10^{-11} M. This was strong evidence that the recombinant receptor was indeed functional in signal transduction. Nevertheless, it was still possible that all it was really doing was serving to bind very large amounts of IL-1, in effect greatly raising the local cell surface concentration of IL-1 seen by the endogenous hamster receptors, and that the hamster receptors were the ones that were actually mediating the signal transduction.

In order to address this issue we made another construct. We introduced a translational stop codon just inside the transmembrane region, so that it produced a molecule which is inserted in the membrane normally and has an intact extracellular ligand binding portion but has deleted almost the entire cytoplasmic domain. When CHO cells stably transfected with this construct and expressing about 80,000 IL-1 binding sites per cell were assayed for their response to IL-1, they completely failed to show an increase in sensitivity. In fact, they behaved similarly to control CHO cells transfected with the expression plasmid carrying no insert. This is conclusive evidence that the recombinant IL-1R itself is actually capable of mediating signal transduction, and is the only molecule that we need to introduce into the CHO cells in order to greatly increase their sensitivity to IL-1.

Signal Transduction of IL-1 and IL-1R

I'm not going to describe a lot about the mechanism by which signal transduction is mediated by the recombinant receptor, in part because we haven't done many experiments in that area, in part because the article of Mizel *et al.* in this volume (Chapter 1) describes one mechanism by which IL-1 may mediate its effects. Based on the sequence of the IL-1R, it is clear that it is not a protein kinase. It lacks many of the standard protein sequence motifs that are characteristic of all tyrosine or serine/threonine protein kinases. We also have found no evidence in standard direct phosphorylation experiments that the IL-1R is a kinase. However, it is clear that one of the early events that happens in response to IL-1 is that a number of cell proteins get phosphorylated. One of these is the IL-1 receptor itself (15). Experiments involving a dose response curve measuring the level of the phosphorylation in response to increasing amounts of IL-1 resulted in that maximal phosphorylation of the IL-1R is reached at levels of IL-1 that would be sufficient to occupy only five percent of the cell surface IL-1R.

This is an extremely interesting finding because it may explain a puzzling phenomenon regarding IL-1, namely that it has a very large so-called "spare receptors effect." What that means essentially is that there is a significant displacement between the biological response curve to IL-1 and the physical binding curve. For example, the T cell lymphoma LBRM produces IL-2 in response to IL-1 stimulation, with a threshold level of about 10^{-14} M IL-1. IL-2 production plateaus at about 10^{-12} M IL-1. However, at this level very few of the IL-1R on these cells are actually occupied. Significant levels of receptor occupancy are not seen until about 10^{-10} M IL-1 (16). This phenomenon has been very puzzling, and in fact has caused a few people to postulate the existence of a second IL-1R of substantially higher affinity than that which described in this chapter even though such a receptor has never actually been seen. However, beyond the fact that the cloned IL-1R molecule, with an affinity constant of about 3×10^9 M^{-1} for IL-1, is capable of mediating biological responses to very low IL-1 concentrations in the CHO transfectants, we can now actually put forth a model to explain why IL-1 is so potent in signalling.

What we imagine is that when IL-1 binds to a receptor on the surface of a cell, that causes in some way a change in the conformation of the cytoplasmic part of the receptor molecule. This in turn leads to activation of a protein serine/threonine kinase that then phosphorylates a variety of substrates, among which is the IL-1R. But it phosphorylates not only the IL-1R molecules that have actually bound IL-1 with their extracellular portions, but in addition phosphorylates many other IL-1R molecules that have not actually interacted with IL-1. We suggest that this may convert those unoccupied receptors to a form which is active in signalling. If this is the case, then it would take very low fractional occupancy of the IL-1R in order to lead to the maximum biological response to IL-1. This sort of model would account for the tremendous amplification that is seen in IL-1 responsive systems. At the moment, of course, this is purely a model, but there are experiments that we can do to test it and those experiments are in progress at the present time.

IL-1R on T Lymphocytes

We have cloned the human IL-1R using cross-hybridization to the mouse IL-1R cDNA (17). The two molecules are very similar. Both have extracellular domains of 319 amino acids, and signal peptide, transmembrane and cytoplasmic regions of similar length. In terms of sequence, the cytoplasmic domains are the most similar with 78 percent amino acid identity, and the transmembrane domains the most dissimilar (although still fairly closely related at 48 percent amino acid identity). One might speculate, based on the great similarity between the cytoplasmic domains in the mouse and human IL-1R, that they have not diverged very much because of a need to maintain interaction with a second protein such as a kinase, but that is pure hypothesis.

The next point to make about the human IL-1R is that, unlike the IL-1R expressed in murine T cells, the IL-1R on the human T cell clone we have used shows a curvilinear Scatchard plot. That is, there are two different affinity classes of IL-1R present on these cells. The major class of receptors has an affinity constant of about 5×10^9 M^{-1}, which is the same as that as of the receptors found on EL 4 cells. The other class of IL-1R, which constitutes about ten percent of the total, has an affinity for IL-1 which is about two orders of magnitude higher than that of the majority class. We have no idea what the difference is between the two affinity classes of receptor, whether it involves interaction with another protein molecule or simply a different state of protein aggregation. We have shown that the lower affinity class of receptors is perfectly capable of mediating signal transduction in response to very low concentrations of IL-1. When the human IL-1R$^+$ T cell clone is transfected into COS cells, it generates a biphasic Scatchard plot. It recreates the two affinity classes of IL-1R seen on the human T cells, even though the COS cells have been transfected with a single cDNA molecule.

Heterogeneity of IL-1R

The receptor that I have described in this article is the major, if not the only IL-1R expressed in T cells and also in fibroblasts. We know further that it is expressed in hepatocytes and keratinocytes, although we don't know whether or not there may be other types of IL-1R expressed in those cells as well. But there are other cell types, the best characterized being B cells, whose IL-1R appears to be the product of a different gene altogether (18, 19). First, crosslinking experiments using the murine pre-B cell leukemia line 70Z/3 show a receptor of about 65 kd in size, in contrast to the 80 kd receptor found on T cells and fibroblasts. The receptor found on EBV-transformed human B cells is also in the range in the range of 60 to 68 kd. Second, while there is substantial binding of radioactive IL-1α to 70Z/3 cells, there is no binding whatsoever of a monoclonal antibody raised against the IL-1R expressed in EL 4 cells. From independent experiments we have reason to believe that this antibody reacts with protein and not with carbohydrate determinants. Therefore, its lack of reactivity on the 7OZ/3 cell would suggest that the extracellular portions of the two IL-1R are different.

A third experiment addresses the similarity of the cytoplasmic portions of the B cell and T cell IL-1R. The IL-1R on the 7OZ/3 pre-B cells shows a curvilinear Scatchard plot. Both affinity classes of IL-1R are down modulated rapidly in response to phorbol esters. The IL-1R on EL 4 cells, however, does not change in its level of surface expression after either 15 minutes or four hours of exposure to to phorbol esters. This suggests that the intracellular portions of the receptors are different.

Finally, using the T cell type IL-1R as a probe in Northern blots, we have been unable to find any RNA in the 7OZ/3 cells that corresponds to mRNA species found in T cells and fibroblasts for IL-1R. In addition, in screening several million cDNA clones derived from the 7OZ/3 pre-B cell line under various stringency conditions, we have been completely unable to find anything which cross-hybridizes in a meaningful fashion with the T cell IL-1R probe. We conclude that the IL-1R molecules expressed in B and T cells differ in both their extracellular and in their cytoplasmic portions, and that those differences reflect not simply post-translational modification but actually expression of two entirely different genes which are dissimilar enough that they don't cross-hybridize at the nucleic acid level.

ACKNOWLEDGEMENTS

This work was supported by a joint venture between Immunex Corporation and Sterling Drug Inc.

REFERENCES

1. Namen, A. E., Schmierer, A. E., March, C. J., Overell, R. W., Park, L. S., Urdal, D. L., and Mochizuki, D. Y. (1988): *J. Exp. Med.* 167:988-1002.
2. Namen, A. E., Lupton, S., Hjerrild, K., Wignall, J., Mochizuki, D. Y., Schmierer, A., Mosley, B., March, C. J., Urdal, D., Gillis, S., Cosman, D., and Goodwin, R. G. (1988): *Nature (London)* 333:571-573.
3. Conlon, P. J., Morrissey, P. J., Jordan, R. P., Grabstein, K. H., Prickett, K. S., Reed, S. G., Goodwin, R., Cosman, D., and Namen, A. E. (1989): *Blood* 74:1368-1373.
4. Watson, J. D., Morrissey, P. J., Namen, A. E., Conlon, P. J., and Widmer, M. B. (1989): *J. Immunol.* 143:1215-1222.
5. Morrissey, P. J., Goodwin, R. G., Nordan, R. P., Anderson, D., Grabstein, K. H., Cosman, D., Sims, J., Lupton, S., Acres, R. B., Reed, S. G., Mochizuki, D., Eisenman, J., Conlon, P. J., and Namen, A. E. (1989): *J. Exp. Med.* 169:707-716.
6. Dower, S. K., Kronheim, S. R., March, C. J., Conlon, P. J., Hopp, T. P., Gillis, S., and Urdal, D. L. (1985): *J. Exp. Med.* 162:501-515.
7. Dower, S. K., Kronheim, S. R., Hopp, T. P., Cantrell, M., Deeley, M., Gillis, S., Henney, C. S., and Urdal, D. L. (1986): *Nature* 324:266-268.
8. March, C. J., Mosley, B., Larsen, A., Cerretti, D. P., Braedt, G., Price, V., Gillis, S., Henney, C. S., Kronheim, S. R., Grabstein, K., Conlon, P. J., Hopp, T. P., and Cosman, D. (1985): *Nature* 315:641-646.
9. Sims, J. E., March, C. J., Cosman, D., Widmer, M. B., MacDonald, H. R., McMahan, C. J., Grubin, C. E., Wignall, J. M., Jackson, J. L., Call, S. M., Friend, D., Alpert, A. R., Gillis, S., Urdal, D. L., and Dower, S. K. (1988): *Science* 241:585-589.
10. Dower, S. K., Wignall, J. M., Schooley, K., McMahan, C. J., Jackson, J.L., Prickett, K. S., Lupton, S., Cosman, D., and Sims, J. E. (1989): *J. Immunol.* 142:4314-4320.

11. Priestle, J. P., Schar, H. P., and Grutter, M. G. (1988): *EMBO J.* 7:339-343.
12. Sims, J. E., and Dower, S. K., unpublished data.
13. Fanslow, W. C., Sims, J. E., Sassenfeld, H., Morrissey, P. J., Gillis, S., Dower, S. K., and Widmer, M. B. (1989): (Submitted).
14. Curtis, B. M., Gallis, B., Overell, R. W., McMahan, C. J., deRoos, P., Ireland, R., Eisenman, J., Dower, S. K., Sims, J. E. (1989): *Proc. Natl. Acad. Sci. (USA)* 86:3045-3049.
15. Gallis, B., Prickett, K. S., Jackson, J., Slack, J., Schooley, K., Sims, J. E., and Dower, S. K. (1989): *J. Immunol.* 143:3235-3240.
16. Dower, S. K., Call, S. M., Gillis, S., and Urdal, D. L. (1986): *Proc. Natl. Acad. Sci. (USA)* 83:1060-1064.
17. Sims, J. E., Acres, R. B., Grubin, C. E., McMahan, C. J., Wignall, J. M., March, C. J., and Dower, S. K. (1989): *Proc. Natl. Acad. Sci. (USA)* (in press).
18. Bomsztyk, K., Sims, J. E., Stanton, T. H., Slack, J., McMahan, C. J., Valentine, M. A., and Dower, S. K. (1989): *Proc. Natl. Acad. Sci. (USA)* 86:8034-8038.
19. Chizzonite, R., Truitt, T., Kilian, P. L., Stern, A. S., Nunes, P., Parker, K. P., Kaffka, K. L., Chua, A. E., Lugg, D. K., and Gubler, U. (1989): *Proc. Natl. Acad. Sci. (USA)* 86:8029-8033.

Molecular Aspects of Immune Response and Infectious Diseases, edited by H. Kiyono, E. Jirillo, and C. DeSimone. Raven Press, Ltd., New York, © 1990.

5

Lymphokine Receptor Signal Transduction and Regulation of Lymphokine Genes

J. Schreurs*, K. Sugimoto*, H. -M. Wang*, J. Nishida*, T. Heike*, S. Miyatake*, E. Abe*, J. Ninomiya-Tsuji*, M. Muramatsu*, N. Ito*, D. Gorman*, K. Maruyama*, G-x. Xie*, T. Kitamura*, K. Hatake*, K. Hayashida*, R. de Waal Malefijt*, J. Shlomai+, N. Ito*, T. Yokota*, K. Arai‡, A. Miyajima* and N. Arai*

*Department of Molecular Biology, DNAX Research Institute of Molecular and Cellular Biology, Palo Alto, California 94304, USA; +Hadassah Medical School, Kuvin Center for the Study of Infectious and Tropical Diseases, Jerusalem, Israel; and ‡Department of Molecular Biology, The Institute of Medical Science, University of Tokyo, 4-6-1 Shirokanedai, Minato-ku, Tokyo, Japan.

IL-3 RECEPTOR AND CELLULAR RESPONSES

The immune response, initiated by exposure to foreign antigens, results in the release of a variety of lymphokines and cytokines (1, 2). With their growth-, differentiation- and function-enhancing properties, lymphokines can rapidly expand lymphocytic and hemopoietic cell populations. The nature of the immunologic response may in part be controlled by a limited diversity in T cell types, each of which produce distinctive patterns of lymphokines. However, the final scenario of the immunologic reaction is governed by the nature of the responding cells, i.e., the presence and absence of specific membrane receptors, the type(s) of signal transduction events, and the presence of specific repertoires of proteins unique to the cell's function. Thus for example, IL-3 is directly stimulatory for mast and myeloid cell growth (3), but has no effect on the peritoneal macrophage, and yet it can act in synergy with macrophage-colony stimulating factor (M-CSF) to augment peritoneal macrophage proliferation (4).

Our biochemical studies of cellular responses to lymphokines have focused on the mouse interleukin 3 (IL-3) receptor in the mast cell-like lines, IC2 and MC/9. The IC2 cell line is responsive to IL-3, granulocyte/macrophage-colony stimulating factor (GM-CSF), and IL-4 whereas, MC/9 cells respond to IL-3 and IL-4. Recently, Kitamura et al. (5) established an IL-3-, GM-CSF-, erythropoietin-

and/or IL-5-dependent human cell line called, TF1. The multiplicity of lymphokines able to stimulate proliferation in the MC/9, IC2, and TF1 cells provides an opportunity to dissect out common elements of the signal transduction pathways for cell survival and proliferation.

IL-3 Receptor Structure - Cross-Linking, Antibodies, and Expression Cloning

As structure determines function, we were interested in biochemically and pharmacologically describing the membrane proteins responsible for IL-3 binding and signal transduction. Previous investigations had indicated that the mouse IL-3 receptor was a low abundance, high affinity (K_D=50-300 pM) molecule of 70-75 kD (6-8). However, through cross-linking assays (9, 10), monoclonal antibodies (11), sucrose density centrifugation (12), affinity chromatography (13) and expression cloning (14), we and others find that a molecule of high molecular mass also binds IL-3.

In addition to the previously described high affinity receptor [K_D=100-300 pM; slow rate of dissociation (k_{-1}=2.7 x 10^{-3} min^{-1})], we also find a second, 10-fold more abundant low affinity (K_D=10-20 nM) site with a rapid rate of dissociation (k_{-1}=0.116 min^{-1}) (9). In cross-linking experiments, we identified the low affinity ^{125}I-IL-3 binding moiety, as two bands of 115 and 140 kD (corrected for the binding of a single 20 kD IL-3) which were a) not saturated at concentrations of 10-30 nM ^{125}I-IL-3 and b) found to have a rapid dissociation rate ($T_{1/2}$=2 min; 4°C) upon addition of excess unlabeled IL-3 immediately prior to the cross-linking.

The human IL-3 receptor appears similar to the mouse receptor in that it is a low abundance, high affinity site with slow dissociation kinetics. Is there a second, low affinity binding site? In some cells, Park *et al.* (15) have seen binding of two different affinities. The size of the human receptor is similar to that of the mouse, proteins of 140 and 70 kD have been cross-linked by IL-3 (16). A major difference between the mouse and human receptors exists in the apparent ability of human IL-3 to compete with GM-CSF (and vice versa) for binding; mouse IL-3 and GM-CSF are specific for their respective receptors. Park *et al.* (15) proposed that a unique binding site with capacity to recognize both IL-3 and GM-CSF exists. Recent data by Scheffler (personal communication) indicates that IL-3 competition for the GM-CSF receptor occurs only in cell lines expressing high affinity GM-CSF receptors and not in cell lines expressing low affinity receptors. Thus, a potential alternative model explaining this data would suppose that intra-receptor cross-talk or competition for a common subunit may regulate lymphokine binding.

The recent production of monoclonal antibodies to the IL-3 receptor has provided independent verification of the structure, composition, and functions of the receptor. One monoclonal antibody to the IL-3 receptor was derived from spleen cells of a non-injected autoimmune MRL/lpr mouse (17). This antibody specifically competes ^{125}I-IL-3. It also is an agonist, mimicking IL-3, e.g., stimulating the tyrosine kinase and cell growth (11); this may occur either through an anti-idiotypic route or by cross-linking of high affinity receptors. A second antibody, AIC-2, recently derived and characterized by Yonehara *et al.* (18) appears to recognize the low affinity form of the receptor. It precipitates a 105 kD molecule, which is able to bind ^{125}I-IL-3 to form complexes of M_r 140 and 90 kD.

We cloned the IL-3 receptor by expression in COS 7 cells and screening with the monoclonal antibody AIC-2 (15). Interestingly, the cloned molecule (M_r = 115 kD) has the characteristics of the low affinity binding site described above, and as

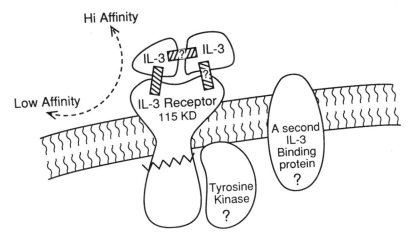

FIG. 1. A schematic of the structure of the IL-3 binding protein and its relationship to the tyrosine kinase.

summarized in Figure 1, lead us to propose the following working model. First, a) the low affinity IL-3 binding moiety is a single entity of M_r 115 kD, b) degradation of this protein gives rise to a 70 kD product, and c) cross-linking of a dimer of IL-3 may give rise to an apparent 140 kD molecule. Second, what molecule(s) comprises the high affinity binding site? Since a small percentage of the ^{125}I-IL-3 bound to the 115 and 140 kD molecules is stable to washing or challenge with unlabeled IL-3, the high and low affinity binding molecules may both contain gp115, alternately a second, distinct high affinity molecule may exist. Third, we show an associated tyrosine kinase, its nature is at this time unclear.

Signal Transduction

The primary proliferative signal induced by IL-3 may be mediated by a tyrosine kinase. However, it is important to recognize that the intracellular signals generated by IL-3 may be multiple. Thus, there is also evidence that IL-3 stimulates the phosphorylation of serine and threonine residues (19), the actions of phosphoglycerol-dependent serine/threonine kinase (20), and the translocation of protein kinase C (PKC) (21). Intriguingly, the stimulation of PKC may occur by a mechanism distinct from the known phosphotidylinositol pathway, as several groups have been unable to demonstrate any IL-3 mediated phosphoinositide hydrolysis (22). It remains to be shown how these discrete biochemical pathways interact.

A variety of evidence links an IL-3 activated tyrosine kinase with the signal transduction pathway responsible for cell survival and proliferation. IL-3-dependence can be abrogated by oncogenes having a tyrosine kinase, such as v-abl or v-src (23, 24). Moreover, expression in IL-3 dependent cells of a mutant v-abl carrying a temperature-sensitive tyrosine kinase renders this IL-3 dependence temperature-sensitive (10, 25). Tyrosine phosphorylation is a direct consequence of IL-3 interaction with its receptor. Using different polyclonal antibodies, proteins phosphorylated at tyrosine residues were detected independently by either immunoprecipitation or Westerns. By immunoprecipitation, a membrane-bound, ^{32}P-labeled 150 kD molecule was detected only after cell stimulation with IL-3, but not with IL-4 or GM-CSF (26). Tyrosine phosphorylation was induced by IL-3 within a minute, suggesting a close link between receptor and kinase. In contrast, Western blotting revealed a radically different set of IL-3-induced tyrosine-phosphorylated proteins (11, 27) of M_r 160, 95, 90, 70, 58, and 50 kD. IL-4 weakly stimulated the phosphorylation of two molecules of M_r 170 and 110 kD. Interestingly, the signal transduction mechanism of GM-CSF may be more similar to IL-3 than previously supposed; human neutrophils also have a GM-CSF-responsive tyrosine kinase which phosphorylates proteins of M_r 140, 95, 75, and 40 (28).

Receptor Transfection Studies

Upon activation by a specific ligand, growth factor receptors initiate a cascade of intracellular signals which ultimately lead to DNA synthesis and cell division. Although the initial stimuli provided by different growth factors may vary, the basic machinery for DNA replication should be the same in all cell types and signals induced by different growth factors may merge. To examine this assumption, we asked whether an unrelated growth factor receptor, having a tyrosine kinase, the epidermal growth factor (EGF) receptor, could trigger cellular responses in an IL-3 dependent cell line.

Transfection using a retroviral vector led to the stable integration and expression of the EGF receptor in the premast cell-like line, IC2 (29). The receptors bind with both high and low affinity and EGF stimulation elicits a short term growth response, yet EGF is unable to maintain long term cell proliferation. Interestingly, a combined incubation with IL-3 and EGF causes cell differentiation into more mature mast cells, as characterized by increased histamine content and intracellular granulation. This differentiation is reversible upon the removal of EGF. Moreover, the consequences of EGF receptor expression in transfectants differ depending on the cellular background. Thus, 32D myeloid cells, transfected and selected for expression of the EGF receptor, were EGF-dependent in long term assays and became more granulocytically differentiated (30).

What are the potential intracellular signalling pathways for the differentiative effect? It is known that EGF induces phosphoinositide hydrolysis and increases cytosolic Ca^{2+} (31); whereas IL-3 has been shown to activate C kinase without increasing the turnover of inositol phospholipids (22). However, since phorbol-12-myristate-13-acetate (PMA) only partially substitutes for IL-3, this suggests that additional signals are required for long-term IL-3 dependent growth. To investigate the putative roles of these various signalling pathways in IC2 cell differentiation, we examined the effects of various activators, such as PMA and A23187. We found that the IL-3/EGF combination was the most efficacious, but treatments with the combination PMA/A23187 or EGF/A23187 also elicited differentiation, indicating possible roles for Ca^{+2} flux and C kinase (29).

Cell Variants: Tools for Delineating Biochemical Pathways

In contrast to T and B cells, it is still not clear whether factor-dependent myeloid cells have a resting G_0 stage. *In vitro*, myeloid cell lines proliferate indefinitely given a source of growth factor, but remove the factor, and the cells die within 24-48 hr.

To better understand the role of IL-3 in the regulation of cell survival and proliferation we have isolated a mast cell mutant, IC2-2, that survives IL-3 depletion by entering G_0/G_1 (32). In the presence of IL-3, there are no detectable differences between the mutant and parental cells. The derivation of such a mutant, in which only the survival of the cell is affected, suggests a separation between the regulatory signals necessary for maintenance and proliferation. Enhanced production of cellular oncogenes such as c-myc, has previously been correlated with cellular proliferation. In the mutant IC2-2 cells, we find that c-myc expression is correlated with cell survival rather than with cell growth, as: 1) c-myc levels were stable in the resting mutant; 2) c-myc declined prior to cell death; and 3) IL-3 stimulation of growth in the mutant had no effect on c-myc. This model is supported by the results of Dean *et al.* (33) in which the constitutive expression of a recombinant retrovirus carrying a c-myc gene rescues the FDCP-1 cell line from death consequent to removal from IL-3.

T CELL ACTIVATION SIGNALS REGULATE THE LYMPHOKINE GENES

Helper T cells produce a battery of lymphokines upon antigenic stimulation (1, 2). The activation of T cells is triggered by binding of an antigen to the T cell receptor/CD3 complex. This activation is mimicked by anti-CD3 antibodies or by treatment with phorbol ester and calcium ionophore (PMA/A23187) (34). All of these various activation signals stimulate PKC and enhance calcium influx (35). Using a mutant PKC which is constitutively active, we have recently shown that in Jurkat cells, the mutant kinase is able, with the addition of exogenous calcium ionophore, to activate the interleukin 2 gene (36). Events downstream of the PKC activation are still unclear, yet the signal must be transmitted to the nucleus to activate transcription. In this review, we focus on the final event of the signal transduction cascade, i.e., the transcriptional regulation of lymphokine genes.

Activation of Lymphokine Genes by PMA/A23187, p40[tax] and E2

Using transient transfection assays in Jurkat cells, we have shown that several lymphokine genes are activated either by PMA/A23187 or virus-encoded transactivators, such as BPV-E2 and HTLV-I p40tax (37, 38). The E2 protein is known to activate the BPV enhancer through a direct binding to the consensus sequence ACCNNNNNNGGT (39). Interestingly, a C-terminally truncated E2 protein retained its capacity to activate the GM-CSF gene (40), suggesting that an E2 protein-protein interaction occurs rather than a direct binding of E2 to DNA.

Sequence analysis of genomic clones revealed no striking homologies among the lymphokines although the 5'-upstream sequences were well conserved between species. However, a conserved decanucleotide (5'-GAGATTCCAC-3') sequence, which we termed the conserved lymphokine element 1 (CLE1), is found in the 5' flanking region of several lymphokine genes (38). Another conserved sequence, CLE2 (5'-TCAGGTA-3'), as well as a GC box exist in the 5' flanking region of the IL-3 and GM-CSF genes (41).

The element of the GM-CSF gene which responds to PMA/A23187, E2 or p40[tax] was mapped by deletion analysis (38, 40). The region mediating the response is at positions -113 to -73 and contains three DNA motifs: CLE1, CLE2 and the GC box. CLE2 and the GC box (positions -95 to -73) are able to confer responsiveness to PMA/A23187, p40^{tax} and E2 (38), whereas, the CLE1 motif (positions -113 and -95) can respond to p40^{tax} but not to E2 or PMA/A23187 stimulation. Thus, the final target site in normal T cell activation is likely the CLE2/GC region, and the CLE1 motif is only the target site for p40^{tax}.

Binding Proteins at the CLE2/GC Box

To characterize the binding proteins which recognize the CLE2/GC box, we carried out gel retardation assays with nuclear extracts from either un-stimulated or PMA/A23187-stimulated Jurkat cells. As shown in Figure 2, four to five retarded bands were detected in the non-stimulated extract using a synthetic oligonucleotide probe which covers the CLE2/GC region. Three of them (A1, A2 and B) were specific to this region as shown by competition assays (42). Additional bands were detected in a PMA/A23187-stimulated extract and are called Nuclear factor of GM-CSF 2 (NF-GM2).

To determine the sequence requirement for NF-GM2 binding, one-base-substituted mutant oligonucleotides were employed in competition assays. Mutations in the CLE2 motif as well as, mutations outside (at positions -85 and -83, Figure 5) did not permit competition for NF-GM2 binding (42), suggesting that NF-GM2 may recognize the region encompassing both CLE2 and the GC box. As previously described (38), the CLE/GC region has homology to the NFκB site, found in the immunoglobulin κ enhancer sequence (43). Interestingly, a SV40 enhancer sequence containing the NF-κB binding site confers PMA/A23187 responsiveness to the proximal GM-CSF promoter region (downstream of -60) (38). Furthermore, the fact that the NF-κB sequence competes for binding to the NF-GM2 complex (42) strongly suggests that the inducible factor, NF-GM2 is identical to NF-κB or is one of a family of NF-κB-like proteins.

Stimulation of T cells by PMA/A23187 may ultimately cause activation of CLE2/GC box through the activation of NF-GM2 binding protein(s). To examine whether this same factor, NF-GM2, also mediates the p40^{tax} or E2 signals, we prepared nuclear extracts from p40^{tax} transformed Jurkat cells and carried out gel retardation assays with CLE2/GC sequence as a probe. As shown in Figure 2, the NF-GM2 complex was detected in the absence of PMA/A23187 stimulation. These results strongly suggest that NF-GM2 is the common transacting factor which mediates the response to both T cell activation signals and p40^{tax}.

Function of NF-GM2 in an *In Vitro* Transcription Assay

To investigate the function of NF-GM2 in transcription, we have established an *in vitro* transcription system, which is stimulation dependent. Transcriptionally active nuclear extracts were prepared from non-stimulated and PMA/A23187-stimulated Jurkat cells. Run-off assays used a GM-CSF promoter template covering the upstream sequence up to -96. As shown in Figure 3, PMA/A23187-stimulated extracts give higher transcriptional activity than non-stimulated extracts and the initiation site of transcription *in vitro* is the same as *in vivo* (42, 44). Moreover, the transcriptional activity in the stimulated extract, as well as in the non-stimulated extract, is CLE2/GC-dependent (42).

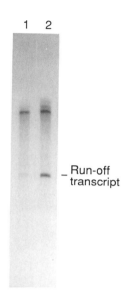

FIG. 2. DNA binding proteins which recognize CLE/GC region 32-P labeled oligonucleotides containing CLE2/GC region positions between -96 and -73 was used as a probe. Protein-DNA complexes were separated from free-DNA probe by native polyacrylamide gel. Each nuclear extract (10 mg/ml proteins) from non-stimulated, PMA/A23187-stimulated or p40[tax] stably-transformed Jurkat cells was titrated.

A Model for GM-CSF Gene Activation in Jurkat Cells

On the basis of these results, we present a model describing how the GM-CSF gene is activated subsequent to T cell stimulation (Figure 4). Downstream of the T cell antigen receptor complex, a multi-step process requiring a series of protein-protein interactions, such as the activation of PKC (36) culminates in the activation of the lymphokine genes. At the end of this cascade, a sequence-specific DNA binding protein, NF-GM2, interacts with CLE2/GC box of the GM-CSF promoter in an inducible manner. Viral transactivators, e.g., p40[tax] or E2, interact with NF-GM2 or with another factor which then activates NF-GM2.

Regulation of IL-3 Gene Expression

IL-3 is expressed almost exclusively by helper T cells activated by antigen or lectin, but is also expressed in mast cell lines, in response to high affinity Fcε receptor stimulation as described in detail in Chapter 2 (45). An abnormal insertion of enhancer elements upstream of the IL-3 gene also leads to constitutive

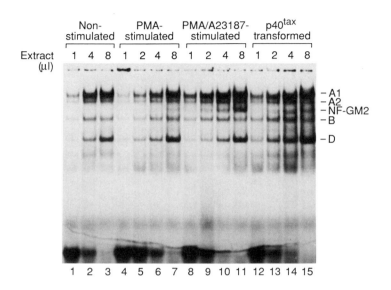

FIG. 3. *In vitro* run-off transcription assay with non-stimulated and PMA/A23187-stimulated extracts. Run-off transcription with GM-CSF template containing the CLE2/GC region (up to -96) was carried out with non-stimulated and PMA/A23187-stimulated extracts. The arrow indicates the run-off transcript.

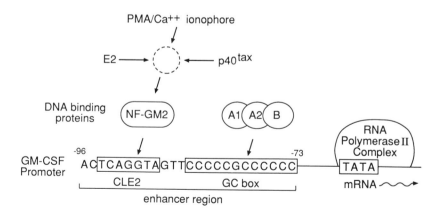

FIG. 4. A possible model for the activation of the GM-CSF gene.

expression of IL-3, as seen in the WEHI-3B cell line (46) or some human lymphoblastic leukemias of B-cell lineage with translocations of chromosome 5 (47). A human T cell line, Jurkat, expresses IL-3 as well as GM-CSF and IL-4, in response to PMA/A23187.

The human IL-3 gene consists of 5 exons and 4 introns (48) and is tandem to and 5' upstream of, the GM-CSF gene (49). Similar to the GM-CSF gene (see above), the 5' upstream region of the human IL-3 gene contains several characteristic sequences, CLE1, CLE2 and a GC rich region at positions between -127 and -49. To investigate the role of these elements, the 5' flanking region of IL-3 was fused to the bacterial CAT or firefly luciferase genes. The fusion plasmids were introduced into Jurkat cells, expressed transiently, and stimulated with PMA/A23187 or by co-transfection of p40^{tax}. The GC rich region at positions -76 to -65 (Figure 5A) responded to p40^{tax} stimulation and it also responded weakly to PMA/calcium ionophore when the more sensitive luciferase assay was used, whereas both CLE1 and CLE2 were dispensable. Moreover, this GC rich region, which is homologous to the GC-box of the human GM-CSF gene (at positions -72 to -64 of human GM-CSF), also enhances TAT-box dependent transcriptional activity *in vitro* (upstream-dependent transcription). A gel retardation assay shows that several proteins bind to this GC-rich region, one of which is induced by PMA/A23187 stimulation. Our results also suggest that the basic IL-3 promoter lacking an upstream region is transcribed efficiently *in vitro* if the region downstream of TATA box at positions between -30 and -17 is intact. It appears that the IL-3 gene does not have a specific enhancer element, but may instead be regulated by a distant enhancer, such as that of GM-CSF.

Regulation of IL-4 Expression

The production of IL-4 is restricted to T cells. In mouse cell lines, IL-4 is produced only by T_H2 cells but not by T_H1 cells, which instead produce IL-2 and IFN-γ. In order to identify cis-acting sequences essential for IL-4 gene regulation, luciferase constructs with various lengths of 5'-upstream human IL-4 (huIL-4) sequence were transfected into Jurkat cells. The huIL-4 gene containing the 176 bp sequence upstream from the CAP site responds to p40^{tax} and E2, viral transactivators, as well as, PMA/A23187. Transfection into the B21 cell line, an human T cell clone, as well as an HTLV-1 transformed T cell clone provided confirmation of this observation. No additional enhancer activity was found in the region other than the 5' upstream region of IL-4 gene. Further analysis identified an 11 bp sequence (P-region: -79 to -69 of huIL-4) as the minimum sequence conferring PMA/A23187 responsiveness to the basic promoter. Interestingly, as shown in Figure 5B, the P-region does not share any homology with the IL-2 promoter, even though surrounding sequences share 84% homology between IL-2 and IL-4 (IL-2: position -91 to -66 versus IL-4: position -91 to -80, and -67 to -53). Moreover, Site-A (position -89 to -73 of human IL-2 gene), which is recognized by the NF-IL-2A protein(s), was identified as one of the essential regions for IL-2 gene expression (50). Thus, characterization of the binding protein(s) which recognizes the P-region and comparison with the NF-IL-2A proteins(s) may provide important clues toward an understanding of the molecular basis of differential regulation between T_H1 and T_H2 T cells.

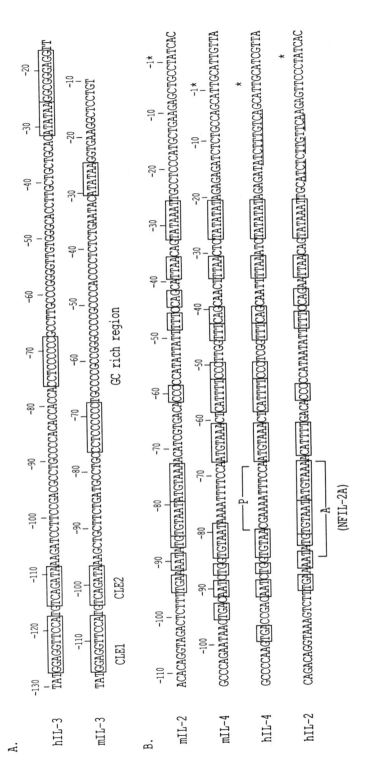

FIG. 5. A; Regulatory region of the IL-3 gene (49, 51). B; Comparison of regulatory region of IL-4 and IL-2 genes (52,53,54,55).

SUMMARY

Much progress has been made in our understanding of the structure of the IL-3 receptor. IL-3 binding occurs through interactions with either a high or a low affinity receptor. Biochemical analysis, monoclonal antibodies, and expression cloning of the low affinity receptor show it to be a molecule of 115 kD, with no tyrosine kinase domain. A definition of the interrelationship between the high and low affinity receptors and the tyrosine kinase awaits further biochemical characterization. To analyze the regulation of lymphokine genes, we have: 1) delineated the *cis*-acting regulatory elements of the GM-CSF and IL-3 genes, which respond *in vivo* to T-cell stimulatory signals; 2) characterized the DNA binding proteins that interact with these *cis*-elements and; 3) established an *in vitro* transcription system which is dependent on the *cis*-regulatory elements. These studies will set the stage for the definition of the transacting factors, which are found downstream of protein kinase C in the T cell activation pathway.

REFERENCES

1. Arai, K., Yokota, T., Miyajima, A., Arai, N., and Lee, F. (1986): *BioEssay* 5:166-171.
2. Miyajima, A., Miyatake, S., Schreurs, J., DeVries, J., Arai, N., Yokota, T., and Arai, K. (1988): *FASEB J.* 2:2462-2473.
3. Rennick, D. M., Lee, F., Yokota, T., Arai, K., Cantor, H., and Nabel, G. J. (1985): *J. Immunol.* 134:910-914.
4. Chen, B. D. M., and Clark, C. R. (1986): *J. Immunol.* 137:563-570.
5. Kitamura, T., Tange, T., Terasawa, T., Chiba, S., Kuwaki, T., Miyagawa, K., Piao, Y., Miyazono, K., Urabe, A., and Takaku, F. (1989): *J. Cell. Physiol.* 140:323-334.
6. Palaszynski, E. W., and Ihle, J. N. (1984): *J. Immunol.* 132:1872-1877.
7. Park, L., Friend, D., Gillis, S., and Urdal, D. L. (1986): *J. Biol. Chem.* 261:205-210.
8. Nicola, N. A., and Peterson, L. (1986): *J. Biol. Chem.* 261:12384-12389.
9. Schreurs, J., Arai, K., and Miyajima, A. (1989): *Growth Factors* 2:221-234.
10. Miyajima, A., Schreurs, J., Wang, H. M., Maruyama, K., Gorman, D., Koyasu, S., Yahara, I., Wang, J., Ohta, Y., and Arai, K. (1989): In: *The Fourth International Congress on Immunopharmacology*, edited by J. W. Hadden, F. Spreafico, Y. Yamamura, K. F. Austen, P. Dukor, and D. Masek, pp. 87-93, Pergamon Press, New York.
11. Schreurs, J., Sugawara, M., Arai, K., Ohta, Y., and Miyajima, A. (1989): *J. Immunol.* 142:819-825.
12. Isfort, R. J., Stevens, D., May, W. S., and Ihle, J. N. (1988): *J. Biol. Chem.* 263:19203-19209.
13. Mui, A. L. -F., Sorensen, P. H. B., Kay, R. J., and Krystal, G. (1989) In: *Hemopoiesis*, Vol. 120, edited by D. Golde, and S. Clark, (in press), Alan R. Liss, New York.
14. Itoh, N., Yonehara, S., Schreurs, J., Gorman, D., Maruyama, K., Ishii, A., Yahara, I., Arai, K., and Miyajima, A. (1990): *Science* (in press).
15. Park, L. S., Friend, D., Price, V., Anderson, D., Singer, J., Prickett, K. S., and Urdal, D. L. (1989): *J. Biol. Chem.* 261:205-210.
16. Kuwaki, T., Kitamura, T., Tojo, A., Matsuki, S., Tamai, Y., Miyazono, K., and Takaku, F. (1989): *Biochem. Biophys. Res. Comm.* 161:16-22.
17. Sugawara, M., Hattori, C., Tezuka, M., Tamura, S., and Ohta, Y. (1988): *J. Immunol.* 140:526-530.
18. Yonehara, S., Ishii, A., Yonehara, M., Koyasu, S., Miyajima, A., Schreurs, J., Arai, K., and Yahara, I. (1989): *Int. Immunol.* (in press).
19. Evans, S. W., Rennick, D., and Farrar, W. L. (1986): *Blood* 68:906-913.
20. Klemm, D. J., and Elias, L. (1988): *Exp. Hematol.* 16:855-860.
21. Farrar, W. L., Thomas, T. P., and Anderson, W. B. (1985): *Nature* 315:235-237.
22. Whetton, A. D., Monk, P. N., Consalvey, S. D., Huang, S. J., Dexter, T. M., and Downes, C. P. (1988): *Proc. Natl. Acad. Sci. USA* 85:3284-3288.

23. Pierce, J. H., DiFiore, P. P., Aaronson, S. A., Potter, M., Pumphrey, J., Scott, A., and Ihle, J. N. (1985): *Cell* 41:685-693.
24. Watson, J. D., Eszes, M., Overell, R., Conlon, P., Widmer, M., and Gillis, S. (1987): *J. Immunol.* 139:123-129.
25. Kipreos, E. T., and Wang, J. Y. (1988): *Oncogene Res.* 2:277-284.
26. Koyasu, S., Tojo, A., Miyajima, A., Akiyama, T., Kasuga, M., Urabe, A., Schreurs, J., Arai, K., Takaku, F., and Yahara, I. (1987): *EMBO J.* 6:3979-3984.
27. Morla, A., Schreurs, J., Miyajima, A., and Wang, J. Y. J. (1988): *Mol. Cell. Biol.* 8:2214-2218.
28. Gomaez-Cambronero, J., Yamazaki, M., Metwally, F., Molski, T. F. P., Bonak, V. A., Huang, C. K., Becker, E. L., and Sha'afi, R. I. (1989): *Proc. Natl. Acad. Sci.* 86:3569-3573.
29. Wang, H. M., Collins, M., Arai, K., and Miyajima, A. (1989): *EMBO J.* 12: (in press).
30. Pierce, J. H., Ruggiero, M., Fleming, T. P., DiFiore, P. P., Greenberger, J. S., Varticovski, L., Schlessinger, J., Rovera, G., and Aaronson, S. A. (1988): *Science* 239:628-631.
31. Schlessinger, J. (1988): *Biochem.* 27:3119-3123.
32. Tsuji, N., Miyajima, A., Arai, K., and Matsumoto, K. (1989): (Submitted).
33. Dean, M., Cleveland, J. L., Rapp, U. R., and Ihle, J. N. (1987): *Oncogene Res.* 1:279-296.
34. Weiss, A., Wiskocil, R. L., and Stobo, J. D. (1984): *J. Immunol.* 133:123-128.
35. Nishizuka, Y. (1986): *Science* 233:305-310.
36. Muramatsu, M., Kaibuchi, K., and Arai, K. (1989): *Mol. and Cell. Biol.* 9:831-836.
37. Miyatake, S., Seiki, M., de Waal Malefyt, R. Heike, T., Fujisawa, T., Takebe, Y., Nishida, J., Shlomai, J., Yokota, T., Yoshida, M., Arai, K., and Arai, N. (1988): *Nucl. Acids Res.* 16:6547-6566.
38. Miyatake, S., Seiki, M., Yoshida, M., and Arai, K. (1988): *Mol. Cell. Biol.* 12:5581-5587.
39. Howley, P. (1987): In: *Cancer Cells, Papillomaviruses*, Vol. 5, edited by B. M. Steinberg, J. H. Brandsma, and L. B. Taichman, pp. 1-4, Cold Spring Harbor Laboratory Press, New York.
40. Heike, T., Miyatake, S., Yoshida, M., Arai, K., and Arai, N. (1989): *EMBO J.* 8:1411-1417.
41. Stanley, E., Metcalf, D., Sobieszczuk, P., Gough, N. M., and Dunn, A. R. (1985): *EMBO J.* 4:2569-2573.
42. Sugimoto, K., Miyatake, S., Arai, K., and Arai, N. (1989): (Submitted).
43. Sen, R., and Baltimore, D. (1986): *Cell* 46:705-716.
44. Miyatake, S., Otsuka, T., Yokota, T., Lee, F., and Arai, K. (1985): *EMBO J.* 4:2561-2568.
45. Plaut, M., Pierce, J. M., Watson, C. J., Hanley-Hyde, J., Nordan, R. P., and Paul, W. E. (1989): *Nature* 339:64-67.
46. Ymer, S., Tucker, Q. J., Sanderson, C. J., Hapel, A. J., Campbell, D., and Young, T. G. (1985): *Nature* 317:255-258.
47. Grimaldi, J. C., and Meeker, T. C. (1989): *Blood* 73:2081-2085.
48. Yang, Y. C., and Clark, S. C. (1987): *Molecular Basis of Lymphokine Action* VOL:325-337.
49. Yang, Y. C., Kovacic, S., Kriz, R., Wolf, S., Clark, S. C., Wellems, T. E., Nienhuis, A., and Epstein, N. (1988): *Blood* 71:958-961.
50. Durand, D. B., Shaw, J. -P., Bush, M. R., Replogle, R. E., Belagaje, R., and Crabtree, G. R. (1988): *Mol. Cell. Biol.* 8:1715-1724.
51. Miyatake, S., Yokota, T., Lee, F., and Arai, K. (1985): *Proc. Natl. Acad. Sci. USA* 82:316-320.
52. Otsuka, T., Villaret, D., Yokota, T., Takebe, Y., Lee, F., Arai, N., and Arai, K. (1987): *Nucl. Acids Res.* 15:333-344.
53. Arai, N., Nomura, D., Villaret, D., DeWaal Malefijt, R., Seiki, M., Yoshida, M., Minoshima, S., Fukuyama, R., Maekawa, M., Kudoh, J., Shimizu, N., Yokota, K., Abe, E., Yokota, T., Takebe, Y., and Arai, K. (1989): *J. Immunol.* 142:274-282.

54. Fujita, T., Takaoka, C., Matsui, H., and Taniguchi, T. (1983): *Proc. Natl. Acad. Sci. USA* 80:7437-7441.
55. Fuse, A., Fujita, T., Yasumitsu, H., Kashima, N., Hasegawa, K., and Taniguchi, T. (1984): *Nucl. Acids Res.* 12:9323-9331.

Molecular Aspects of Immune Response and Infectious Diseases, edited by H. Kiyono, E. Jirillo, and C. DeSimone. Raven Press, Ltd., New York, © 1990.

6

Intercellular Communication: Macrophages and Cytokines

C. A. Nacy, S. J. Green, D. L. Leiby, B. A. Nelson, R. M. Crawford, A. H. Fortier, D. L. Hoover, and M. S. Meltzer

Department of Cellular Immunology, Walter Reed Army Institute of Research, Washington, DC 20307-5100, USA

The immune response functions principally as an amplification system: a very small change in homeostatic balance elicits a local response that rapidly escalates to a systemic reaction, and tissue integrity is eventually restored. The principal cells involved in the initiation and resolution of immune reactions are macrophages and lymphocytes. The amplification process is bidirectional: macrophages instruct lymphocytes that an event has occurred, lymphocytes proliferate and, in turn, recruit more macrophages to restore homeostasis. Intercellular communication between these cells occurs through the synthesis, release, and recognition of small molecular weight (8-70 kD) glycoproteins, called cytokines. These cytokines have many characteristics that are similar to hormones of the endocrine system. Unlike hormones, however, that are produced in one organ to act on cells in distant organs, cytokines are produced, and act, locally at the site of neoplastic or infectious insult.

Immunologists have been analyzing biological activities of cytokines *in vitro* for over 20 years. With the advent of molecular cloning techniques, there are now dozens of cytokines available as single reagents to test for function *in vivo* and *in vitro*. Some cytokines appear to have restricted activities; some have many activities, and affect a variety of cell types. Then again, certain effector activities can only induced by, or are greatly enhanced by, the treatment of cells with a series of cytokines. The key question for immunologists today is not only which cytokines are involved in the resolution of disease, but when do these cytokines function, and which of their many *in vitro* activities are important *in vivo*. Clearly, the single cell / single cytokine / single activity theory of cellular interaction underestimates the potential impact of a cytokine on cells in its environment.

Our approach to immunoregulatory cytokines is to view these molecules as the language of the immune system: words for intercellular communication. The task of immunologists, like linguists, is to unravel the complexities of this language. That different cells use different symbols for induction of the same activity (for example, IL-2 by T_{H1} cells, IL-4 by T_{H2} cells, for induction of T cell growth) suggests that there may even be dialects or regional differences based on class of cells. Further, in our own language, the meaning of a word in a sentence changes with the context in which the word is spoken. Thus modifying phrases become important for clarity. The same is true for cytokines: the sequence of cytokines is very important for interpretation by cells in an immune reaction, as well. In this paper, we review briefly three major concepts that have evolved from the study of intercellular communication over the last few years: redundancy, synergy, and cooperation.

REDUNDANCY: DIFFERENT CYTOKINES INDUCE THE SAME ACTIVITY

Redundance is quite common in nature: the genetic code and gene duplication are but two obvious and well known examples. Once single cytokines are tested

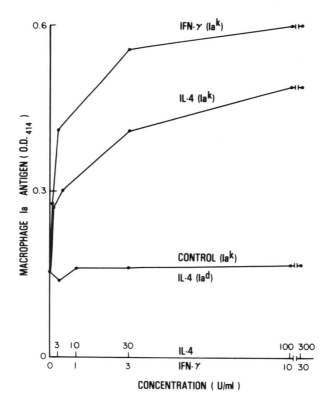

FIG. 1. Treatment of macrophages from C3H/HeN mice (Ia^k) with IFNγ or IL-4 for induction of Ia antigens.

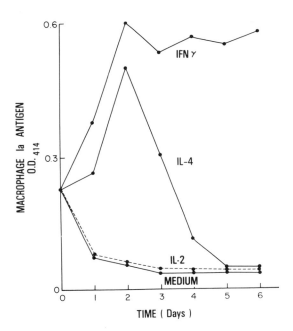

FIG. 2. Kinetics of Ia expression by macrophages treated with IFNγ or IL-4.

for activities other than those by which they were originally defined, it becomes clear that redundancy is the rule rather than the exception in immunoregulation, as well. TNFα and IL-1 share several activities; IL-2 and IL-4 both act as T cell growth factors; IFNγ and TNFα regulate similar effector activities; and IL-4 and IFNγ have multiple overlapping activities on macrophages. For example, macrophages treated with either IL-4 or IFNγ for 24 hr express Ia antigen, an essential component of antigen presentation during induction of immune reactions (1) (Figure 1). Analysis of the induction of Ia, however, demonstrated profound differences in the regulation of this macrophage antigen by the two lymphokines. The kinetics of macrophage Ia expression showed a peak of activity at 24 hr for both IFNγ and IL-4; Ia expression induced by IFNγ remained at maximal levels for over 96 hr, while Ia expression induced by IL-4 returned to baseline levels by 48 hr (Figure 2). When Ia-specific mRNA was examined in these cells by dot blot analysis, message for Ia persisted in IFNγ-treated cells, while both mRNA and protein decreased to baseline in IL-4 treated cells.

Additionally, these lymphokines appear to regulate Ia expression in different cell populations. IFNγ induces Ia antigen on roughly 75-80% of treated macrophages; IL-4 induces expression of Ia on only 30-40% of macrophages from the same population. Combined treatment with IFNγ and IL-4 showed that the effects were additive over a broad dose response. Thus, two distinct lymphokines have overlapping activities for induction of macrophage Ia, but appear regulate these activities in distinct subpopulations of cells. It is interesting to note that the two lymphokines are produced by different subpopulations of helper T cells, as well. Why might there be redundancy in lymphokine activities? Perhaps these lymphokines operate at different *in vivo* sites, or at different times during an immune response. In any case, the number of cytokines reported to have similar activities on cells is increasing daily.

SYNERGY: ACTIVITY OF ONE CYTOKINE IS ENHANCED BY THE PRESENCE OF A SECOND CYTOKINE

A number of years ago, we demonstrated the synergistic interaction of lymphokines and bacterial lipopolysaccharides (LPS) (2). While LPS had no effect on the induction of macrophage tumoricidal activity itself, addition of small amounts of LPS markedly enhanced the activity of lymphokines for induction of this effector activity. More recently, we examined the effect of LPS on the activation of macrophages for tumoricidal and microbicidal activity by a variety of recombinant cytokines. We found that certain cytokines could induce these effector reactions by themselves, but LPS greatly potentiated the activity of each of the active cytokines (Figure 3). It is interesting to note that LPS did not make an inactive cytokine active in either of the two assays.

A number of recent studies show synergy with different cytokine combinations: IL-1 augments NK-cell activity induced by IFNγ (3); TNFα enhances IFNγ activation of human neutrophils (4), and monocyte / macrophages (5) for tumoricidal activity; and synergistic toxic effects on tumor cells are reported for IFNγ and lymphotoxin (6-8). Synergy, then, is another method of amplification in immune reactions.

COOPERATION: NO SINGLE CYTOKINE IS EFFECTIVE, BUT TWO (OR MORE) TOGETHER CAN INDUCE THE ACTIVITY

Induction of activated macrophage resistance to infection can only be accomplished by the interaction of several lymphokines (9, 10). If cells are treated with IFNγ and either IL-2, IL-4 or GM-CSF they resist infection with the protozoan parasite, *Leishmania major*, as well as several other obligate or facultative intracellular parasites (Figure 4).

What sets this reaction apart from synergistic interactions described above is that no single cytokine can induce the effector function. IFNγ is, however, an essential component of the reaction cascade: treatment of cells with any other combination of cytokines, such as IL-2 and IL-4, or IL-2 and GM-CSF, is not effective. Despite the absolute necessity for IFNγ in the reaction mixture, the sequence of cytokine interaction with the cell is unimportant. Thus cells treated with IFNγ first, then IL-2, or visa versa, develop equivalent resistance to infection. In addition, unlike tumoricidal activity and intracellular killing (Figure 3), LPS does not augment the expression of this effector activity by cells treated with single cytokines, or cells treated with single cytokines in the presence of IFNγ (10). So the activity of IFNγ and the different cytokines for induction of activated macrophage resistance to infection is not synergy, but cooperation.

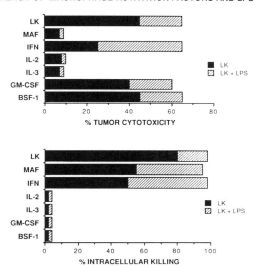

FIG. 3. Synergistic activity of LPS for cytokine-induced tumoricidal activity (fibrosarcoma TU-5) and microbicidal activity (*Leishmania major* amastigotes).

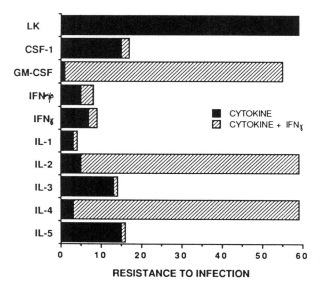

FIG. 4. Cooperation of lymphokines for induction of macrophage resistance to infection with *Leishmania major* amastigotes.

We analyzed in some detail the cooperative interaction of IFNγ and IL-2, principally because the concept of IL-2 as a macrophage activation factor is rather novel. The activation of macrophages by these two cytokines actually involves a third cytokine produced by the macrophage itself: TNFα. If we treat macrophages with IFNγ and IL-2 for 20 hr, then add soluble antibodies to TNFα into the reaction mixture of activated macrophages and parasites, we totally abrogate the expression of resistance to infection (Table 1). Whether TNFα serves as the proximal effector molecule for destruction of the parasite, or is simply the third cytokine in a sequence that induces another, unknown effector molecule, is not yet clear. It is interesting that cells activated by another combination of cytokines, IFNγ and IL-4, are not affected by the presence of anti-TNFα antibodies. Thus there must be at least two different mechanisms that result in the same phenotypic expression of the effector reaction.

TABLE 1. Inhibition of Macrophage Resistance to Infection by Rabbit Anti-Mouse TNFα Polyclonal Antibody

Macrophages Treated With:	% Infected Macrophages	% Resistance To Infection
Medium	34 ± 3	0
Anti-TNFα Ab	31 ± 5	9
IFNγ	30 ± 6	12
IL-2	26 ± 3	6
IL-2 + IFNγ	18 ± 5	47
IL-2 + IFNγ + Anti-TNFα Ab	30 ± 3	12

CELLS TALKING TO CELLS

We've only just begun to discover the activities of different immunoregulatory cytokines, and have, at this point, no real concept of how these cytokines function *in vivo*. Still, the advances made by the endocrinologists studying hormone function, and biochemists studying intracellular regulatory events, each incredibly complex systems, are encouraging. We started with the single cell / single cytokine / single activity theory of immunoregulation, and are progressing tentatively to more complex theories: one small step at a time. The anticipated breakthrough in deciphering the language of intercellular communication will be both time and energy-dependent: when the disparate findings of a number of investigators, both *in vitro* and *in vivo*, begin to fit a pattern, we will have taken that giant step. Even before we have our own corner of intercellular communication reasonably organized, we are faced with the real possibility that immunoregulatory cytokines and endocrine hormones do not function exclusively in their own areas: the number of neuroendocrine effects on immune cells that are reported in the literature is increasing exponentially. Considering the complex nature of tissues, and the variety of insults available to upset homeostasis, it is no wonder that regulatory systems are redundant, highly reactive, and very interactive.

REFERENCES

1. Crawford, R. M., Finbloom, D. S., Ohara, J., Paul, W. E., and Meltzer, M. S. (1987): *J. Immunol.* 139:135-141.
2. Ruco, L. P., and Meltzer, M. S. (1978): *J. Immunol.* 121:2035-2042.
3. Dempsey, R. A., Dinarello, C. A., Mier, J. W., Rosenwasser, L. J., Allgretta, M., Brown, T. E., and Parkinson, D. R. (1982): *J. Immunol.* 129:2504-2510.
4. Shalaby, M. R., Aggarwal, B. B., Rinderknecht, E., Swedersky, L. P., Finle, B. S., and Palladino, M. A. (1985): *J. Immunol.* 135:2069-2073.
5. Philip, R., and Epstein, L. B. (1986): *Nature (London)* 323:86-89.
6. Stone-Wolff, D. S., Yip, Y. K., Kelker, H. C., Le, J., Henriksendestefano, D., Rubin, B. Y., Rinderknecht, E., Aggarwal, B. B., and Vilcek, J. (1984): *J. Exp. Med.* 159:828-843.
7. Williams, T. W., and Bellanti, J. A. (1983): *J. Immunol.* 130:518-520.
8. Lee, S. N., Aggarwal, B. B., Rinderknecht, E., Assisi, F., and Chiu, H. (1984): *J. Immunol.* 133:1083-1086.
9. Davis, C. E., Belosevic, M., Meltzer, M. S., and Nacy, C. A. (1988): *J. Immunol.* 141:627-635.
10. Belosevic, M., David, C. E., Meltzer, M. S., and Nacy, C. A. (1988): *J. Immunol.* 141:890-896.

Molecular Aspects of Immune Response and Infectious Diseases, edited by H. Kiyono, E. Jirillo, and C. DeSimone. Raven Press, Ltd., New York, © 1990.

7

Nerves, Neuropeptides and the Regulation of the Mucosal Immune Response

J. Bienenstock, M. G. Blennerhassett, K. Croitoru, P. B. Ernst, J. Gauldie, M. Jordana, J. S. Marshall, M. H. Perdue, A. M. Stanisz, and R. H. Stead

Department of Pathology, Molecular Virology and Immunology Programme, and Intestinal Diseases Research Unit, McMaster University, Hamilton, Ontario, Canada, L8N 3Z5

INTRODUCTION

It has been known for many years that mucosal immune mechanisms differ in several respects from those which characterize non-mucosal organs, including blood. It is well established that local immune reactions may occur without any reflection of these events in the circulation. In this paper, we present our thoughts on how nerves and neuropeptides might modulate the local microenvironment at mucosal surfaces, and thus partake in the inflammatory response. Before this, however, we will provide some background information on mucosal immunity. The reader is referred to reviews published elsewhere for details and references (1-7).

IgA

Mucosal tissues are characterized, by the predominance of secretory IgA in secretions, which is reflected by a predominance of IgA synthesizing lymphocytes in the interstitial tissues. Most mucosal epithelia have the capacity to selectively transport dimeric IgA into the secretions. In the rat gastrointestinal tract, the majority of the IgA found in the secretions is not synthesized in the immediate vicinity, but appears there by virtue of selective transport by hepatic parenchymal cells from the circulation into the biliary tract, and thence to the intestine. The secondary minor IgA component is locally synthesized by lymphocytes in the lamina propria. The extent to which local synthesis contributes to the presence of

IgA in secretions differs in different tissues, and also among species. In consideration of the transport of dimeric IgA across epithelia, the factors which regulate the cellular secretory process itself may play a significant role in the amount of immunoglobulin found in external secretions, independent of factors which regulate the immune system itself. Such factors may include hormones generated locally or at distant sites.

Antigen Processing

Antigen processing is initiated by the follicle associated epithelium covering the specialized lymphoid follicles found in the mucosa of the respiratory and gastrointestinal tracts. The function of the rest of the mucosal epithelium in handling and processing antigen as a part of an immune response, is by no means clear. However epithelium, especially that which is involved in inflammatory events, expresses Ia antigens, and it is clear that the epithelium can be involved in immune processing.

Lymphocyte Traffic

The number of immunoglobulin containing cells in a given tissue depend on the type and location of the tissue, as well as the bacterial, viral or antigen load, and such things as gender and hormal status. The lymphocytes in most of these tissues appear to be derived from the circulation, and a variety of factors regulate cellular delivery to the tissues and their subsequent extraction from the blood. These include age, the state of the vascular endothelium, the blood flow, the presence of specific antigen in local tissues, the general nutritional state and dietary intake.

Lymphocytes derived from mucosal tissues, upon subsequent reinjection, tend to selectively localize in the tissue of origin, and secondarily in other mucosal tissues, in preference to systemic lymphoid tissues. The basis for these observations is still under discussion, but has been incorporated into a general concept of a common mucosal immune system. The initiation of the mucosal immune response may therefore occur in the mucosal lymphoid follicles, in the epithelium, lamina propria and interstitium, or in the draining lymph nodes. There is evidence in support of all of these mechanisms being involved, to a greater or lesser extent.

T Cell Regulation of IgA Production

There has been much written about the T cell regulation of IgA synthesis (see details in Chapter 8 by McGhee *et al.*). There is general agreement that IgA is a T cell-dependent isotype, in that interleukins 2, 3, 4 & 6 may contribute individually to its synthesis or synergize to promote differentiation from an IgA bearing cell to one which synthesizes and secretes this molecule. Another type of T cell which may be responsible for the switch of immunoglobulin synthesis to the IgA isotype, has been postulated. Increasing evidence suggests that T cells may also be responsible for contrasuppressive effects, and that these systems may be isotype specific (including IgA).

Intraepithelial Leukocytes (Lymphocytes)

A population of leukocytes often referred to as intraepithelial leukocytes or lymphocytes (IEL) exist within mucosal epithelia. In the mouse, these cells (of which about 60% contain granules) do not bear the pan-T phenotypic marker Thy 1, but do possess CD8 positivity. Recently, this population has been shown to be CD3+, and express γδ T-cell antigen receptors on their surface. A closer examination of the cellular function of IEL has revealed that they possess a high precursor frequency for mast cells, the presence of cytotoxic T cell precursors as well as cytotoxic T cells, cells responsible for antibody dependent cellular cytotoxicity and natural killer (NK) activity. In addition, cells with the capacity to specifically kill certain virus infected targets have been identified. When estimates have been made as to which of these activities are dependent on cells expressing classical T cell markers, the majority are found in this biologically characterized population; the 60% of IEL which comprises the granulated CD8+, CD3+ cells are still left as a functional enigma without any defined biological activity.

Mast Cells

In the last decade it has become clear that mast cells are heterogeneous in terms of growth factor dependency, phenotype, proteoglycan content and serine esterases. The phenotype of mast cells has been best characterized in rats, although similar properties have been described to a variable extent in other species. The intestinal mucosal mast cell (IMMC), which is similar to that referred to as the bone marrow derived mast cell, is primarily IL-3 dependent for proliferation, and is characterized by its granular content of chondroitin sulfate di-B and rat mast cell protease II (RMCP II). The connective tissue mast cell (CTMC) may in part be IL-4 dependent, and contains heparin and RMCP I. While these two phenotypes are distinguishable as extremes of the scale, there may be gradations in between. There is clear evidence that each phenotype has the capacity, in the right microenvironment, of being transformed into the other. As will be seen later, the role of the microenvironment may be crucial in the determination of cellular differentiation, and it may play a central role in the regulation of mucosal immune responses.

Nerves

There is a large amount of nervous tissue within mucosal tissues. Furness and Costa have calculated that there are as many nerve cell bodies (10^8) within the gastrointestinal tract as are contained within the whole spinal cord (8). In addition to enteric nerves of the cholinergic and adrenergic types, there are a variety of non-adrenergic, non-cholinergic nerves, many of which are characterized by the presence of peptide neurotransmitters, including substance P (SP), somatostatin (SOM), vasoactive intestinal polypeptide (VIP) and calcitonin gene related peptide (CGRP). Many of the nerves contain multiple neurotransmitters. SP, for example, is often found in sensory afferent nerves in association with CGRP. Nerves are distributed throughout mucosal tissues, often with branches to the epithelium (in the respiratory tract) and capillaries, and with innervation of smooth muscle. The mucosal lymphoid structures are innervated, as are all lymphoid tissues.

NEUROPEPTIDES AND IMMUNITY

One of the first steps in cell activation is the interaction between surface membrane receptors and activating factors. Therefore, it was logical to assume that if neuropeptides were to affect lymphocyte populations, these effects should be mediated via specific receptors. Indeed, it is now well established that such receptors exist and are functional. For example, receptors for VIP have been extensively studied on both human and murine lymphocytes and were shown to be predominantly present on T cell (9, 10). We have shown the presence of SP receptors on murine T and B lymphocytes (11). Similarly, Payan and colleagues described SP receptors on human peripheral blood lymphocytes and several lymphatic cell lines (12). Recently, receptors for SOM were characterized on both murine and human lymphatic cell lines, supporting earlier observation with freshly isolated cells (13). Kinetic analysis and enumeration of specific receptors or binding sites should be approached carefully. Receptor expression is usually dependent on the stage of cell cycle, and different (sometimes very fast) internalization rates. The fact that there is usually a low density of receptors for neuropeptides, as for colony stimulating factors, makes numerical analysis difficult.

The best evidence so far for receptor presence comes from functional studies. Macrophages, when stimulated with SP release PGE_2 and superoxide (14) and lymphocyte function can be significantly altered by SOM, VIP and SP (5). In our studies, neuropeptides either inhibited (SOM and VIP) or enhanced (SP) cell proliferation and immunoglobulin synthesis. Their effects on murine immunoglobulin synthesis was isotype specific: IgA synthesis was mostly affected, IgM and IgG less so. In addition, the neuropeptide effects were organ specific, since cells isolated from Peyer's patches responded to a much greater extent to SP than splenic lymphocytes.

In a series of *in vivo* studies we were able to confirm some of our *in vitro* observations. SP administered *in vivo* over a 7 day period via miniosmotic pumps (ALZA) resulted in an increased serum level of SP of 2-3 fold, and in enhanced cell proliferation and immunoglobulin (IgA>IgM>IgG) production in both Peyer's patches and spleen (5). In an antigen specific system, when sheep red blood cells (SRBC) were used, *in vivo* administration of SP resulted in an enhanced anti-SRBC response. We were also able to demonstrate that SP can significantly alter the NK activity of IEL which are in very close proximity to SP-containing nerves in gut. When incubated *in vitro* with the ^{51}Cr-labeled YAC-1 tumor cells in the presence of SP, the IEL activity was significantly enhanced, compared to controls without SP. Again this effect was organ specific, since IEL but not splenic NK activity was enhanced by SP. The same results were obtained when SP was administered *in vivo* with the ALZA pumps (15).

Other neuropeptides such as VIP, depending on experimental conditions, significantly enhance or suppress the NK activity of human peripheral blood lymphocytes (16). Ottaway has shown that down regulation of VIP receptor expression on murine T lymphocytes affects their ability to selectively localize in mucosal sites (17).

Helme *et al.* have shown that a plaque forming response to SRBC in draining lymph nodes is virtually abolished in neonatally capsaicin treated animals (18). This procedure depletes the animals of SP. When antigen was delivered together with SP in such animals the plaque forming response (both direct and indirect) was restored. The stage of the immune response at which SP is involved is not clear, i.e., the early processing stage, the recruitment of T cells, migration to the lymph nodes or through an undetermined effect on the capillary bed.

Taken together, these observations on the multiple effects of various neuropeptides on immune cells suggest that neuropeptides play an important role as molecular messengers of the nervous system, in the regulation of immune responses. These facts alone provide strong evidence for a link between nervous and immune systems, and their functional as well as anatomical integration.

MAST CELLS AND NERVES

Morphological Evidence of Mast Cell/Nerve Associations

There are numerous reports suggesting a microanatomical association between mast cells and nerves in many tissues (7). We investigated this in detail in the rat and human gastrointestinal mucosae (19, 20). In the rat, 67% of IMMC were closely apposed to neuron specific enolase containing nerves at the light microscopical level. Additionally, SP and CGRP were localized in nerves adjacent to mast cells. In the electron microscope, in animals infected with Nippostrongylus brasiliensis (Nb), which induces mast cell hyperplasia, 8% of the mast cells were found in random sections to have membrane/membrane contact with nerves containing large dense core vesicles, suggestive of peptidergis innervation. In the human intestine we used a combination of PGP9.5 immunohistochemistry and Alcian blue staining, and found between 47% and 78% of IMMC apposed to nerves. Ultrastructural examination of the same cases revealed dilated axonal profiles in direct apposition with mast cell membranes.

Effects of Mast Cells and Nerves on Epithelial Cell Function

The intestinal epithelium has two main functions, that of transport and as a barrier. Transport involves the absorption and secretion of ions, solutes and water; and the barrier function includes the exclusion of potentially pathogenic organisms, and the uptake of macromolecular molecules including antigens. In 1984, Perdue *et al.* showed that perfusion of the jejunum *in vivo* with antigen in sensitized rats produced a decreased net absorption of water, sodium and chloride, with evidence of mast cell degranulation and histamine release (21). Mast cell stabilizing drugs such as doxantrazole prevented this effect, whereas cromoglycate did not, suggesting the involvement of IMMC (22). These antigen dependent effects were shown in Ussing chambers to be due in large part to chloride ion secretion. The effects are mast cell dependent, antigen specific, as well as histamine (H1), serotonin and nerve dependent (23, 24). In addition products of archidonic acid metabolism appear to be involved, and many of the effects have also been attributed to the release of RMCP II, the substrate of which appears to be basement membrane collagen. Since the effects of both luminal and serosal antigen were blocked by tetrodotoxin, a selective nerve blocker, it was interesting that atropine had no effect in this system. Subsequent experiments, in animals treated neonatally with capsaicin, suggested the involvement of SP-containing nerves in this antigen dependent response (23).

Similar experiments have been done in rat lungs *in vivo*, using as a measurement of solute clearance the uptake of a radiolabeled molecular probe $99mTcDTPA$ and subsequent gamma camera computer assisted analysis (25). Aerosolized antigen caused a significant increase in solute uptake, whereas, in neonatally capsaicin treated animals, this was reduced to about 50% of baseline positive control. Ussing chamber experiments on tracheal tissue from sensitized rats again showed a mucosal mast cell, nerve depletion (23). Similar work has now been performed *in vitro* using co-cultured colonic epithelial cells and peritoneal mast cells, and also in tissues from rats, guinea pigs and humans.

These data strongly suggest that mast cells sensitized with IgE or IgG antibodies to specific antigens, communicate with afferent nerves, and through an axon reflex or similar mechanism, act on target epithelial cells to change their function both as transporting and barrier cells.

The Effects of Psychological Conditioning on Mast Cell Function

Because of the apparent nervous involvement in the physiologic systems described above, we have examined the role of classical Pavlovian conditioning on rat mast cell degranulation (26). Rats were sensitized to egg albumin in adjuvants (alum and pertussis) and given a nematode infection to promote IgE synthesis and intestinal mucosal mastocytosis. Conditioning consisted of antigen injections paired with audiovisual cues. Animals were then challenged only with the audiovisual cue. Exposure to the cur alone caused significant serum elevations of the IMMC-specific RMCP II. Subsequent experiments showed, with appropriate negative controls, that conditioned animals exposed to the cue alone had increased baseline chloride ion secretion, supramaximal responses to antigen, and oscillatory bursts of enteric nerve activity blocked by tetrodotoxin (27). Thus the central nervous system (CNS) can directly or indirectly interact with the peripheral nervous system, and cause mast cell degranulation with a number of consequent local mucosal physiological effects.

Interaction of Mast Cells with Nerves in Tissue Culture

There is no information about the early cellular and molecular events that result in the close contacts of mast cells with nerves that are seen in the peripheral nervous system (7). Similarly, there is only indirect evidence that functional interactions occur at these sites. We have recently developed a tissue culture model for the direct investigation of these neterocellular interactions (28). In our studies, isolated sympathetic nerves from the superior cervical ganglia of neonatal mice have been co-cultured, in the presence of nerve growth factor, with either rat basophilic leukemia (RBL) cells, representative of IMMC (29), or with freshly isolated peritoneal mast cells (PMC), typical of CTMC. These sympathetic nerves rapidly formed contacts with RBL, apparently in response to a chemotactic factor (30). These nerve/mast cell contacts were selective, and were maintained for periods of up to 17 hours of continuous observation.

This suggests that nerve/mast cell interactions in culture represent nerve-target cell recognition, involving the development of selective adhesion and possibly the subsequent modification of the nerve to a secreting terminus or varicosity. This is supported by an electrophysiological evaluation which showed that sympathetic nerve contact increases RBL membrane conductance in a manner mimicked only by application of SP but not acetylcholine or nor-adrenaline (30). We interpret this as evidence that functional interactions occurred between these nerves and mast cells in culture.

NERVE GROWTH FACTOR

Nerve growth factor (NGF) was first identified by Levi-Montalcini and colleagues and is a complex of α,β and τ subunits with a sedimentation coefficient of 7S (31). The active nerve growth component is the 2.5S homodimer produced by cleavage of the β subunit, with a molecular weight of 26kDa. There is more than 90% amino acid sequence homology between murine and human NGF. Sympathetic, sensory and cholinergic forebrain neurons are dependent upon NGF for their survival (32, 33) but this differs according to the developmental stage of the animal. Sensory neurons become NGF-independent in the neonatal period; whereas, sympathetic nerves are still NGF-dependent post-natally. In addition to its effects on nerves, NGF may have broader biological functions. For example it has been shown to induce shape changes in platelets and exert chemotactic activity for polymorphonuclear leukocytes. Furthermore, NGF induces mast cell hyperplasia when administered to neonatal rats, which is independent of its action on sympathetic nerves (34). There is also now evidence for the action of NGF on lymphocyte proliferation (35).

NGF Effects on Mast Cells

NGF (2.5S) has been shown to be an extremely potent degranulating agent for rat CTMC both *in vivo* in the skin and for cells derived from the peritoneal cavity *in vitro* (36). This non-cytotoxic event is dependent upon the addition of phosphatidylserine or its lysoderivative *in vitro*. We have recently reported that NGF can also augment antigen or ionophore mediated histamine release from isolated mast cells in the absence of these phospholipids (37). It is known that PMC do not require surface IgE for degranulation to occur in response to NGF, and the mechanism by which NGF acts as a secretagogue remains to be elucidated. Aloe and Levi-Montalcini demonstrated many years ago that injection of 2.5S NGF into neonatal rats induced mast cell hyperplasia (34). In a detailed examination of the NGF induced mast cell hyperplasia *in vivo*, we found that mast cell numbers were increased both in tissues where CTMC are found classically, and in the gut mucosa where IMMC are observed. The greatest relative increase in mast cell numbers was, however, in the hemopoietic spleens of these neonatal animals. Immunohistochemical analysis, using anti-RMCP I for CTMC, and anti-RMCP II for IMMC, demonstrated that despite the significant hyperplasia which had been induced, the phenotype of mast cells observed in any given tissue was not altered (38).

In view of the potent degranulatory ability of NGF, we decided to assess the importance of mast cell degranulation products on the induction of mast cell hyperplasia. NGF was administered to neonatal rats either alone, or in combination with the mast cell stabilizing agent - disodium chromoglycate (DSCG). Concurrent DSCG treatment was found to completely abrogate the NGF induced CTMC hyperplasia. When an alternative CTMC "specific" degranulating agent, compound 48/80, was administered to the neonatal rats, a significant hyperplasia of both CTMC and IMMC was observed. When neonatal animals were given a degranulation supernatant obtained from 98% purified adult rat PMC treated with anti-IgE covalently coupled to Sepharose, a CTMC and IMMC hyperplasia was again induced (39). These results strongly suggest that NGF induces CTMC hyperplasia via an autocrine feedback mechanism. However, NGF induced IMMC hyperplasia may not require mast cell degranulation to occur.

NGF Effects on Colony Growth and Cellular Differentiation

In a human methyl cellulose culture system, we have examined the ability of NGF to affect colony growth. Addition of NGF to peripheral blood cultures in the presence of conditioned medium increased both the total number of colonies and the proportion of Eo-type histamine containing colonies which, on electron microscopy, appear to basophils (40). This effect of NGF was abrogated by the removal of T-cells (by rossetting with SRBC) from the cell population, or by the addition of anti-NGF antiserum. Using the leukemic cell line HL-60, we have found that NGF will synergise with GM-CSF (41) and IL-5, but not IL-3 (42), in inducing histamine containing cells from alkaline passaged butyrate treated cells. This evidence strongly suggests a potential role for NGF in the regulation of hemopoiesis and/or differentiation.

NGF Effects on Lymphocytes

Thorpe, Perez-Polo and colleagues have demonstrated that NGF induces marked but delayed (three to four days) enhancement of DNA synthesis in rat spleen cells cultured with mitogen (35). They have also reported receptors for NGF on rat spleen mononuclear cells, radiolabeled NGF binding to thymocytes (kd=1.5nM) equivalent to that seen with control PC12 cells which express NGF receptors, and the induction of IL-2 receptors' on cultured human lymphocytes (35).

Recently, we have begun to investigate the potential for NGF to act on lymphoid populations by first looking for the NGF receptor immunohistochemically (43). Using a double-staining technique, with monoclonal antibodies 20.4 (anti-NGF receptor) and R4/23 (reacting predominantly with follicular dendritic cells), we have found that the majority of follicular dendritic cells (FDC) express NGF receptor-immunoreactivity in germinal centres in human tonsils, appendix and intestine. The FDC population appears to be heterogenous, however, since in addition to the 20.4+ R4/23+ cells there are also 20.4+ R4/23- and 20.4- R4/23+ dendritic cells in the secondary lymphoid follicles. We have isolated FDC from human tonsils and found NGF receptor immunoreactivity on cells resembling FDC morphologically; and have further purified these cells using magnetic beads (43).

DISCUSSION

There are a multiplicity of potential interactions occurring between structural and other cellular elements of mucosal tissues which may be involved in the regulation of mucosal responses. It may be instructive to examine how these cells and molecules may interact to regulate immunity through a scheme such as that seen in Figure 1.

An immune response initiated somewhere in the body gives rise to an IgE response which would cause the product (IgE) to sensitize mast cells. On subsequent interaction with antigen this results in the release of preformed mediators, and initiates synthesis of new mediators. Many such have been described, but of key interest to this discussion is the recent demonstration that cultured mast cells may synthesize IL-3, -4, -5, -6 and GM-CSF (44, 45) (See Chapter 2 by Ben-Sasson *et al.*). Our recent studies have made it clear that epithelial cells can also make both IL-6 and GM-CSF (46). SP can further promote the epithelial cell synthesis and secretion of IL-6 and will cause activated fibroblasts to synthesize IL-6 and IL-8 (manuscript in preparation). Epithelial cells and fibroblasts can, therefore, no longer be regarded as passive bystanders. Capillary endothelial cells can also synthesize a variety of cytokines including IL-6 and GM-CSF (47, 48) and must also be taken into account in local immune responses. The activation of epithelium, endothelium and fibroblasts may also alter the nature of the extracellular matrix on which the immune-inflammatory response evolves. Different extracellular matrices may differentially bind growth factors such as NGF and GM-CSF and present them to progenitor cells in a biologically active manner. IL-4, -5, and -6 are potent in their recruitment and growth promoting activities for cells of the granulocyte lineage, as well as in the synthesis of both IgA and IgE.

NGF can now be added to the growing list of colony stimulating factors which promote the growth and differentiation of inflammatory cells. Since NGF is synthesized by activated fibroblasts as well as injured nerves (see ref. 5-7), we suggest that this molecule must also be important in local inflammatory events. This may involve activation of mast cells or lymphocytes, the evidence for which we have provided above.

That immune cells can synthesize and secrete peptide neurotransmitters suggests that inflammation might alter the local levels of such substances. Examples of this are the synthesis of bombesin by alveolar macrophages (49) and SP by eosinophils (50). Such molecules might also be released from local nerves or endocrine cells. In turn, this would perturb the events depicted in Figure 1. In this complex and dynamic inflamed environment it is possible that structural or phenotypic changes might also occur in local nerves. It is now known that IL-1 can induce NGF synthesis in sciatic nerve explants (51) and that IL-6 can induce neurite outgrowth from cultured PC12 cells (52). These effects could clearly be integrated into the schema illustrated in Figure 1. Accordingly, we recently looked for changes in the mucosal inervation in rats infected with Nb, which induces marked mastocytosis. In this animal model, about one week after infection, the IMMC degranulate and disappear. We found that this was followed by a two-fold increase in the number of nerves per villus, a four-fold increase in the average nerve cross-sectional area, and a five-fold increase in the nerve area density (53). As the mast cell hyperplasia ensued, the nerve changes subsided. These data suggest that there is increased inervation at some point during the inflammatory response, which might augment the interactions discussed above.

Our conditioning experiments suggest that the CNS might, at least partly, be involved in the modulation of peripheral immunity through the activation of mast cells. In addition to such an efferent action of nerves on mast cells, there is also considerable evidence of mast cell products exciting nerves (see ref. 7). In this respect we believe that mast cell nerve communication may be used as a paradigm of the way in which the nervous and immune systems interact. Clearly, however,

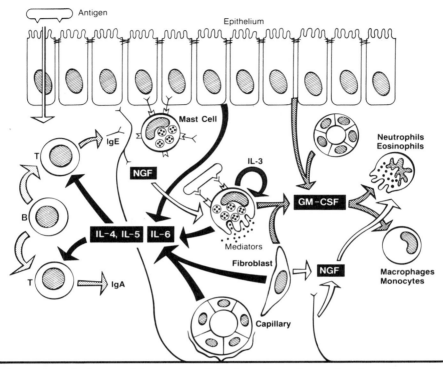

FIG. 1. Schematic diagram of the complex cellular interactions of mucosal surfaces. See text for discussion.

other immune cell types may also be in communication with the nervous system. The evidence in favour of lymphocyte nerve interaction is extensive and reviewed elsewhere (54).

The cellular network involving cytokines, nerves, neuropeptides, and nerve growth factor, while extremely complex, is most interesting. At the very least, this suggests some role for these molecules in the regulation not only of mucosal but other immune responses as well.

ACKNOWLEDGEMENTS

The authors thank MRC Canada and the Council for Tobacco Research (USA) for continued support of this research. Mrs. Bonnie Hugill is also thanked for typing the manuscript.

REFERENCES

1.   Mestecky, J., and McGhee, J. R. (1987): *Advances in Immunology* 40:153-245.
2.   Elson, C. O. (1988): In: *Inflammatory Bowel Disease*, edited by J. B. Kirsner, and R. G. Shorter, pp. 97-164, Lea & Febiger, Philadelphia.

3. Brandtzaeg, P., Sollid, L. M., Thrane, P. S., Krale, D., Bjerke, K., Scott, H., Kett, K., and Rognum, T. O. (1988): *Gut* 29:1116-1130.
4. Ernst, P. B., Befus, A. D., and Bienenstock, J. (1985): *Immunology Today* 6:50-55.
5. Stead, R. H., Bienenstock, J., and Stanisz, A. M. (1987): *Immunol. Rev.* 100:333-359.
6. Stead, R. H., Tomioka, M., Pezzati, P., *et al.* (1989): In: *Psychoneuroimmunology II*, edited by R. Ader, D. L. Felten, and N. Cohen, (in press), Academic Press, Orlando.
7. Stead, R. H., Perdue, M. H., Blennerhassett, M. G., Kakuta, Y., Sestini, P., and Bienenstock, J. (1989): In: *The Neuroendocrine-Immune Network*, edited by S. Freier, pp. 19-37, CRC Press, Boca Raton.
8. Furness, J. B., and Costa, M. (1987): *The Enteric Nervous System*, Churchill Livingstone, New York.
9. Ottaway, C. A., and Greenberg, G. R. (1984): *J. Immunol.* 132:417-423.
10. Danek, A., O'Dorisio, S. M., O'Dorisio, T. M., and George, J. M. (1983): *J. Immunol.* 131:1173-1177.
11. Stanisz, A. M., Scicchitano, R., Dazin, P., Bienenstock, J., and Payan, D. G. (1987): *J. Immunol.* 139:749-754.
12. Payan, D. G., Brewster, D. R., Missirian-Bastian, A., and Goetzl, E. J. (1984): *J. Clin. Invest.* 74:1532-1535.
13. Scicchitano, R., Dazin, P., Bienenstock, J., Payan, D. G., and Stanisz, A. M. (1987): *Brain Behav. Immun.* 1:173-184.
14. Hartung, H. P., Wolters, K., and Toyka, K. V. (1986): *J. Immunol.* 136:3856-3861.
15. Croitoru, K., Ernst, P. B., Bienenstock, J., Padol, I., and Stanisz, A. (1989): (Submitted).
16. Rola-Pleszczynski, M., Boldue, D., and St-Pierre, S. (1985): *J. Immunol.* 135:2569-2573.
17. Ottaway, C. A. (1984): *J. Exp. Med.* 160:1054-1069.
18. Helme, R. D., Eglezos, A., Dandie, G. W., Andrews, P. V., and Boyd, R. L. (1987): *J. Immunol.* 139:3470-3473.
19. Stead, R. H., Tomioka, M., Quinonez, G., Simon, G. T., Felten, S. Y., and Bienenstock, J. (1987): *Proc. Natl. Acad. Sci. USA* 84:2975-2979.
20. Stead, R. H., Dixon, M. F., Bramwell, N. H., Riddell, R. H., and Bienenstock, J. (1989): *Gastroenterology* (in press).
21. Perdue, M. H., Chung, M., and Gall, D. G. (1984): *Gastroenterology* 86:391-397.
22. Perdue, M. H., and Gall, D. G. (1985): *J. Allergy Clin. Immunol.* 76:498-503.
23. Perdue, M., D'Inca, R., Crowe, S., Sestini, P., Marshall, J., and Bienenstock, J. (1989): In *Mast Cell and Basophil Differentiation and Function in Health and Disease*, edited by S. J. Galli, and K. F. Austen, pp. 295-305, Raven Press, New York.
24. Castro, G. A., Harari, Y., and Russell, D. (1987): *Am. J. Physiol.* 253:G540-G548.
25. Sestini, P., Dolovich, M., Vancheri, C., Stead, R. H., Marshal, J. S., Perdue, M., Gauldie, J., and Bienenstock, J. (1989): *Am. Rev. Respir. Dis.* 139:401-406.
26. MacQueen, G., Marshall, J., Perdue, M., Siegel, S., and Bienenstock, J. (1989): *Science* 243:83-85.
27. MacQueen, G., Bienenstock, J., Marshall, J., and Perdue, M. H. (1989): *Gastroenterology* 96:A687.
28. Blennerhassett, M. G., Stead, R. H., and Bienenstock, J. (1987): *Biophysical J.* 51:65A
29. Seldin, D., C., Adelman, S., Austen, K. F., Stevens, R. L., Hein, A., Caulfield, J. P., and Woodbury, R. G. (1985): *Proc. Natl. Acad. Sci. USA* 82:3871-3875.
30. Blennerhassett, M. C., Tomioka, M., and Bienenstock, J. (1989): (Submitted).
31. Levi-Montalcini, R., and Calissano, P. (1986): *Trends in Neurosciences* 9:473-477.
32. Otten, U. (1984): *Trends Pharmacol. Sci.* 5:307-310.
33. Korsching, S. (1986): *Trends in Neurosciences* 9:570-573.
34. Aloe, L., Levi-Montalcini, R. (1977): *Brain Res.* 133:358-366.
35. Thorpe, L. W., Stach, R. W., Morgan, B., Perez-Polo, J. R. (1988): In *Neural Control or Reproductive Function*, edited by J. M. Lakoski, J. R. Perez-Polo, and D. K. Rassin, pp. 351-369, Alan R. Liss, New York.
36. Pearce, F. L., and Thompson, H. L. (1986): *J. Physiology* 372:379-393.
37. Tomioka, M., Stead, R. H., Nielsen, L., Coughlin, M.D., and Bienenstock, J. (1988): *J. Allergy Clin. Immunol.* 82:599-607.
38. Tomioka, M., Stead, R. H., Marshall, J., *et al.* (1989): (Submitted).

39. Marshall, J. S., Stead, R. H., McSharry, C., Nielsen, L., and Bienenstock, J. (1989): (Submitted).
40. Matsuda, H., Coughlin, M. D., Bienenstock, J., Denburg, J. A. (1988): *Proc. Natl. Acad. Sci. USA* 85:6508-6512.
41. Tsuda, T., Dolovich, J., Bienenstock, J., and Denburg, J. (1989): (Submitted).
42. Tsuda, T., Switzer, J., Bienenstock, J., and Denburg, J. (1989): (Submitted).
43. Pezzati, P., Marshall, J. S., Stanisz, A. M., Bienenstock, J., and Stead, R. H. (1989): *Proc. Vth Intl. Congr. Muc. Immunol.* (in press).
44. Plaut, M., Pierce, J. H., Watson, C. J., Hanley-Hyde, J., Nordan, R. P., and Paul, W. E. (1989): *Nature* 339:64-67.
45. Wodnar-Filipowicz, A., Heusser, C. H., and Moroni, C. (1989): *Nature* 339:150-152.
46. Ohtoshi, T., Vancheri, C., Cox, G., *et al.* (1989): (Submitted).
47. Jirik, F. R., Podor, T. J., Hirano, T., Kishimoto, T., Loskutoff, D. J., Carson, D. A., and Lotz, M. (1989): *J. Immunol.* 142:144-147.
48. Bagby, G. C., McCall, E., Bergstrom, K. A., and Burger, D. A. (1983): *Blood* 62:663-668.
49. Wiedermann, C. J., Goldman, M. E., Plutchok, J. J., Sertl, K., Kaliner, M., Johnston-Early, A., Cohen, M. H., Ruff, M. R., and Perx, C. B. (1986): *J. Immunol.* 137:3928-3932.
50. Weinstock, J. V., Blum, A., Walder, J., and Walder, R. (1988): *J. Immunol.* 141:961-966.
51. Lindholm, D., Heumann, R., Meyer, M., and Thoenen, H. (1987): *Nature* 330:658-659.
52. Satoh, T., Nakamura, S., Taga, T., Matsudo, T., Hirano, T., Kishimoto, T., and Kaziro, Y. (1988): *Mol. Cell. Biol.* 8:3546-3549.
53. Stead, R. H., Kosecka-Janiszewska, U., and Bienenstock, J. (1989): (Submitted).
54. Felten, D. L., Felten, S. Y., Bellinger, D. L., Carlson, S. L., Ackerman, K. D., Madden, K. S., Olschowki, J. A., and Livnat, S. (1987): *Immunol. Rev.* 100:225-260.

Molecular Aspects of Immune Response and Infectious Diseases, edited by H. Kiyono, E. Jirillo, and C. DeSimone. Raven Press, Ltd., New York, © 1990.

8

Diversity of Regulatory Mechanisms Required for Mucosal IgA Responses

J. R. McGhee[*], K. W. Beagley[*‡], T. Taguchi[+],
K. Fujihashi[+], J. H. Eldridge[*], C. Lue[*],
Z. Moldoveanu[*], J. Radl[§], J. Mestecky[*+‡] and H. Kiyono[+]

The Departments of [*]Microbiology, [+]Oral Biology and [‡]Medicine, The University of Alabama at Birmingham, UAB Station, Birmingham, AL 35294, USA; and [§]TNO Institute of Experimental Gerontology, Rijiswijk, The Netherlands

INTRODUCTION

Higher mammals possess an immune system which may be divided into two compartments: the internal system consisting of secondary lymphoid tissue such as spleen and lymph nodes, and the immune system of mucosal surfaces. The mucosal immune system has an exceedingly large area to protect, >400 m^2 of wet mucosal membranes of the gastrointestinal (GI), upper respiratory and genitourinary tracts and numerous glandular tissues, e.g., mammary, lacrymal, salivary and other glands (1). The host is well equipped to respond to the myriad of potentially pathogenic microorganisms, allergens, normal flora and foreign antigens which continually impinge upon these surfaces.

The major antibody isotype in external secretions is immunoglobulin A (IgA), and it has been estimated that this Ig class represents > 60% of the total antibodies produced per day in humans (2-4). Further, although IgA in human serum is second in amount to IgG subclasses, the catabolism of IgA is much higher than that of IgG. Therefore, the amount of each isotype produced by the bone marrow, spleen and lymph nodes for the circulatory compartment may in fact be equal (5). More than 98% of the IgA present in external secretions is locally produced by plasma cells in the lamina propria or in the glandular tissues (3). How are immune responses in the external secretions induced and regulated? To answer this question, it is first necessary to describe the unique features of IgA inductive and effector tissues.

IgA INDUCTIVE SITES

We normally inhale or ingest foreign materials and as in other vertebrates, we possess highly developed secondary lymphoid tissues specialized in the sampling of environmental antigens and the regulation of an appropriate secretory IgA (S-IgA) response. The upper respiratory tract contains bronchus-associated lymphoreticular tissues (BALT) which bear morphologic similarities to the tissues present in the GI tract. All mammalian species studied to date possess discrete lymphoid follicles along the wall of the small intestine which are known collectively as gut-associated lymphoreticular tissue, or GALT. GALT consists of Peyer's patches (PP), the appendix, solitary lymphoid nodules (SLN) and an ileocaecal PP (1). The great majority of functional studies with isolated cells have been performed with PP from mice, rats and to a lesser extent rabbits, and the PP are the prototype of an IgA inductive site (1). Mucosal immunologists, assuming that BALT and GALT have similar characteristics and are both major IgA inductive sites, collectively term them mucosal-associated lymphoreticular tissues, or MALT (6).
The structure of the PP includes both a dome region, consisting of lymphocytes, macrophages and small numbers of plasma cells, and a region of underlying follicles (B cell zones) with 1-2 germinal centers and parafollicular areas (T cell zones) (Figure 1). The epithelium covering the dome of the PP is unique in that it contains in addition to columnar cells, cuboidal epithelial cells and a few goblet cells. Because of this, less mucus deterrent is present to impede antigen uptake and lymphocytes lie next to epithelium, which has led to the term *lymphoepithelium* (1). Specialized antigen-sampling cells, termed follicle-associated epithelial (FAE) or microfold (M) cells, occur in this lymphoepithelium (1). FAE or M cells can actively pinocytose proteins or phagocytize particulate antigens, virions or even whole bacteria. Uptake of antigen does not result in degradation in lysosomes, and the intact antigen can reach underlying lymphoreticular cells in the dome region, including antigen-presenting cells. Thus FAE or M cells, in the absence of a mucus layer, serve to sample antigens from the gut lumen. It is unlikely that FAE or M cells actually present antigen in a class I- or II-restricted sense; however, they are important for delivery of antigen to underlying zones where the induction of the immune response takes place.
The follicles of PP contain germinal centers, which are enriched in B cells with surface IgA (sIgA+) (7). Though B cell commitment to IgA synthesis is thought to occur in these sites, developing B cells rarely undergo terminal differentiation into plasma cells there (7, 8). Thus PP are IgA inductive sites and not major effector regions for the synthesis of IgA. GALT contains mature CD3+ T cells, and approximately 60 percent are CD4+ T helper (T_H) cells (Figure 1). Mature CD8+ T cells also are present and both cytotoxic (CTLs) and suppressor (Ts) cells occur in this subset. In addition, CD3+, CD4-, 8- T cells are found which functionally mediate contrasuppression (4).

IgA EFFECTOR SITES

Previous studies in rabbits (9) and more recent ones in mice (reviewed in reference 1), have shown that GALT is the source of precursors of IgA plasma cells that repopulate distant tissues such as the intestines, the mammary, lacrymal, salivary, and cervical glands in the uterus, the respiratory tract, and, to a lesser degree, spleen and lymph nodes. Following primary interaction with antigen in

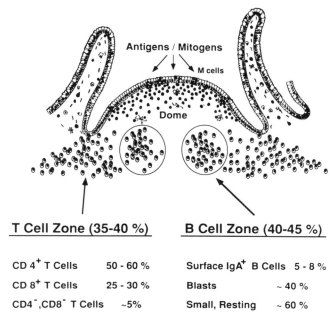

T Cell Zone (35-40 %)   **B Cell Zone (40-45 %)**

CD 4[+] T Cells	50 - 60 %	Surface IgA[+] B Cells	5 - 8 %
CD 8[+] T Cells	25 - 30 %	Blasts	~ 40 %
CD4[−],CD8[−] T Cells	~5%	Small, Resting	~ 60 %

FIG. 1. Illustration of a Peyer's patch (PP) with a lymphoepithelium containing M cells and the underlying dome region. The follicles (B cell zones) contain sIgA[+] B cells, including both activated (blast) and resting populations. The T cell zones contain both CD3[+], CD4[+], Th and CD3[+], CD8[+] cytotoxic/suppressor cells which regulate mucosal responses.

association with PP accessory cells, B and T cells leave the PP via the efferent lymphatics and reach the systemic circulation through the thoracic duct. Circulating B cells then reach and enter distant mucosal tissues where they are preferentially retained (Figure 2). In these mucosal effector sites, B cells clonally expand and then mature into IgA plasma cells (1). Precursor cells containing polymeric IgA (pIgA) with J chain have been found in peripheral blood following oral immunization and are thought to be the migrating population of activated IgA lymphoblasts destined to populate mucosal tissues. Lymphocytes possess specific homing receptors, which mediate binding to the high endothelial cells of postcapillary venules (10); however, a discussion of the mechanisms of lymphocyte recirculation is beyond the scope of this brief review.   The B cells which have migrated into effector sites subsequently differentiate into plasma cells secreting IgA antibodies to the antigen encountered in GALT, resulting in simultaneous production of antibodies in several external secretions. The homing of B cells from GALT and subsequent immunity in mucosal sites have been termed the *Common Mucosal Immune System* (Figure 2) (6, 11).

ROLE OF INTERLEUKINS IN IgA SYNTHESIS

B lymphocytes respond to an array of cytokines which influence their activation, expression of class II MHC and antigen-presenting function as well as control their division and terminal differentiation into Ig-secreting cells. These

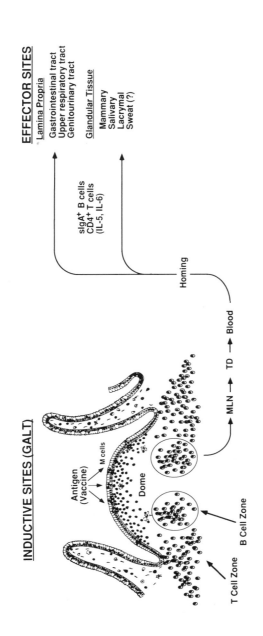

FIG. 2. Model for the induction of S-IgA responses in external secretions via the *Common Mucosal Immune System*. Antigen uptake (by M cells) occurs in GALT and results in the initial induction of the response. Antigen-sensitized, precursor IgA+ B cells and CD4+ Th cells leave via efferent lymphatics and migrate to mesenteric lymph nodes (MLN), and then into the thoracic duct (TD) to the bloodstream. These migrating cells enter the IgA effector sites where terminal differentiation, synthesis and transport of pIgA occurs.

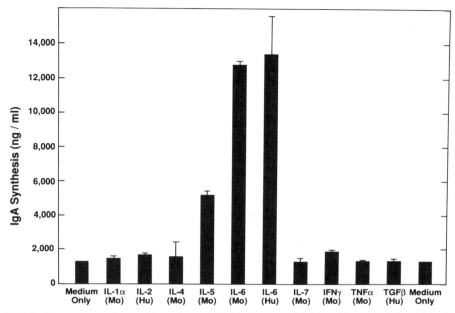

FIG. 3. Comparison of recombinant human (Hu) and mouse (Mo) cytokines for their activity in the induction of IgA synthesis. Appropriate levels of each cytokine were added to cultures of purified PP B cells and the levels of IgA in the supernatants determined 7 days later.

same cytokines affect IgA B cells, and recent studies have suggested that IL-5 and IL-6 (Figure 3) are of particular importance for IgA responses in the murine system (4, 12-18).

IL-5

When added to LPS-driven B cell cultures, purified IL-5 enhanced IgA production, and this effect was further increased by IL-4 (13). Independent studies by others showed that supernatants from T_{H2}-cell clones (see below) enhanced IgA synthesis in LPS-triggered splenic (SP) B cell cultures (14). The IgA-enhancing factor (IgA-EF) was purified from culture supernatants of a T_{H2}-cell clone to apparent homogeneity and shown to be IL-5 (15).

Since the PP possess a high frequency of B cells committed to IgA (Figure 1), recent studies have used PP B cell subsets to measure IL-5-induced effects. It was shown that IL-5 induced-IgA synthesis in LPS-stimulated sIgA+ but not in sIgA- B cells (16). IL-5 also induced increased numbers of IgA-secreting cells but did not enhance cell division in culture, suggesting that IL-5 induces terminal differentiation of IgA-committed (sIgA+) B cells to secrete IgA. A second study (17) in which LPS was used to trigger PP B cells found that IL-5 also induced IgA synthesis in LPS-stimulated sIgA- B cell cultures. However, additional work showed that sIgA+ B cells in PP accounted largely for the IL-5 enhanced response even in the presence of LPS (17).

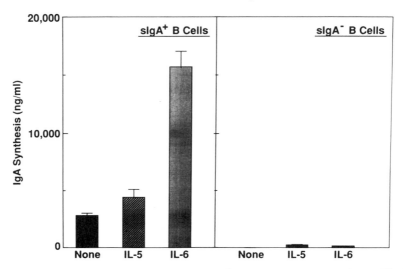

FIG. 4. Effects of rIL-5 and rIL-6 on purified sIgA$^+$ and sIgA$^-$ PP B cell subsets. The PP B cells were purified by panning on anti-Ig plates, stained with FITC anti-α and separated by flow cytometry. Whole PP B and sIgA$^-$ B cells were cultured at 1 x 10^5 cells/well and sIgA$^+$ cells were added at 5 x 10^4 cells/well.

Our group has extensively studied the PP B cell population affected by IL-5 in a system which does not require LPS stimulation. GALT cells are naturally exposed to environmental microbial stimulants, and approximately one-third of PP B cells are in cycle (18). It was thus feasible to separate PP B cells into large blasts and small, resting lymphocytes on Percoll gradients. The addition of recombinant IL-5 (rIL-5) to PP B cell cultures resulted in increased synthesis of IgA, with little or no effect on the IgM or IgG isotypes (Figure 3) (18). The IL-5-induced increase in IgA synthesis was confined largely to the blast sIgA$^+$ B cell subset (Figure 4) and occurred in a dose-dependent fashion (18). Taken together, these studies suggest that IL-5 induces sIgA$^+$ B cells to differentiate into cells secreting IgA in a manner completely analogous to the known effects of IL-5 for other isotypes.

IL-6

It is now well documented that IL-6 induces terminal differentiation of B cells which have been activated with mitogen or antigen (19) (see also Chapter 3 by Kishimoto *et al.*). IL-6 is pleiotropic, and in addition to acting as a B cell differentiation factor, this cytokine also stimulates hepatocytes to secrete acute-phase proteins, induces hematopoietic stem cells, thymocytes, and mature T cells to divide, and acts on other cell types as well (19). Both rIL-5 and rIL-6 induced significant increases in IgA synthesis in PP B cell cultures, while rIL-4 (and other recombinant cytokines) had no effect (Figure 3). In these studies, rIL-6 induced three- to four- fold higher levels of IgA than were seen with rIL-5 (12). Further, rIL-6 induced significant increases in IgA synthesis in cultures of large blast B cells at levels comparable to that induced by rIL-5 in the blast population. When PP B cells were separated into sIgA$^+$ and sIgA$^-$ B cell subsets by flow cytometry, removal of sIgA+ B cells abolished the effect of both rIL-5 and rIL-6 on IgA synthesis (Figure 4). On the other hand, B cells enriched for sIgA+ cells and incubated with rIL-5 or rIL-6 increased IgA synthesis in a dose-dependent manner, with rIL-6 inducing two- to four-fold higher levels of IgA synthesis than rIL-5 (Figure 4). Thus, both IL-5 and IL-6 induce the sIgA+ blast B cell subset to differentiate into IgA-secreting cells.

Since IL-6 induces increased numbers of B cells which secrete IgA and higher levels of total IgA synthesis (12), it is more effective for terminal differentiation than is IL-5. Both IL-5 and IL-6 appear to act on B cells already committed to IgA. Though this finding does not eliminate a possible role for these interleukins in switching, it strongly suggests that they clonally expand IgA-committed precursors to subsequently differentiate into high-rate IgA-secreting plasma cells. Furthermore, this work shows that IL-5 or IL-6 is sufficient to support IgA secretion by cycling sIgA+ PP B cells, without a requirement for additional interleukins or cytokines (Figure 3).

T_{H1} AND T_{H2} CELLS IN GUT-ASSOCIATED TISSUES

Cloned murine CD4+ T_H cells can be divided into two subsets, T_{H1} and T_{H2}, based upon the profile of cytokines they produce (20, 21). T_{H1} cells secrete IL-2, interferon-gamma (IFNγ) and lymphotoxin (TNFβ), while T_{H2} cells produce IL-4, IL-5 and IL-6 (21, 22). It is not yet established whether T_{H1} and T_{H2} cells occur *in vivo* after antigen stimulation; however, it is well known that CD4+ T cells in mucosal sites are in different stages of activation. It would be important to determine if T_{H2} cells occur in gut-associated tissues, since these lymphocytes secrete the interleukins of most importance in IgA synthesis (Figure 3).

To test this, we have developed an enzyme-linked immunospot (ELISPOT) method to allow the detection of individual T cells secreting a particular lymphokine (23). We have used the ELISPOT to detect IFNγ and IL-5-producing cells as illustrated in Figure 5. For the IFNγ assay, the mAbs R4-6A2 and biotinylated XMG1.2 were used in coating and detection, respectively. The mAbs TRFK-5 and biotinylated TRFK-4 were similarly used for enumeration of IL-5 secreting cells (Figure 5). The specificity of the assay was established by use of either cloned Th1 (H66-61) or Th2 (CDC-25) cells, where the T_{H1} produced IFNγ but not IL-5 (Figure 5), while the T_{H2} line produced IL-5 but not IFNγ (Figure 5) (24). Both IFNγ and IL-5 were produced *de novo* since treatment of the T cells with cycloheximide inhibited both IFNγ and IL-5 spot-forming cells (SFC). These results show that the IFNγ and IL-5-specific ELISPOT is a sensitive and specific assay which could be used to determine the frequency of IFNγ- and IL-5-producing cells in gut-associated tissues.

We have assessed the numbers of T cells spontaneously secreting these cytokines in PP, lamina propria lymphocyte (LPL) and intraepithelial lymphocyte (IEL) populations (24). Moderate levels of IL-5 SFC were seen in the IEL subset, while higher numbers occurred in the LPL population. Significant numbers of IFNγ SFC (T_{H1}-type) were also seen in LPLs, but the frequency of IL-5 SFC was always higher (T_{H1}:T_{H2} in LPL=1:3). In IELs, equal numbers of IFNγ and IL-5 SFC were seen. Interestingly, both CD4+ and CD8+ IEL T cells produced these two cytokines. In contrast, T cells freshly isolated from PP, an IgA inductive site, contained fewer IL-5- or IFNγ-secreting cells, while SP T cells had essentially no SFC. When PP or SP T cells were stimulated with Con A, significant and approximately equal numbers of IFNγ- and IL-5-producing cells were seen.

ELISPOT For:	Monoclonal Antibody Used	
	Coating	Detection
IFNγ	R4-6A2	XMG 1.2
IL-5	TRFK-5	TRFK-4

Th Clone	IFNγ SFC	IL-5 SFC
H66-61 (Th1)		
CDC-25 (Th2)		

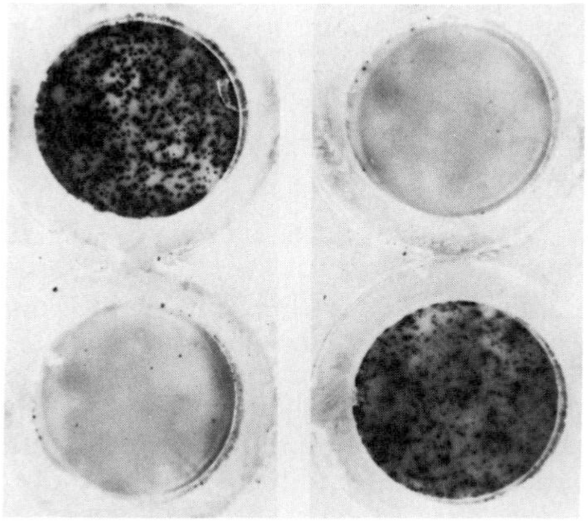

FIG. 5. Protocol for the use of the ELISPOT assay to detect IFNγ and IL-5 producing cells. Nitrocellulose plates were coated with the indicated mAb, and T_{H1} (H66-61) or T_{H2} (CDC-25) clones added. After 20 hr of incubation, the cells were removed and the spots developed with the respective biotinylated mAb, avidin-peroxidase and substrate.

Both IgA inductive (PP) and effector (LPL) sites and the IELs of the intestine contain significant numbers of both IL-5- and IFNγ-producing T cells (24). However, it should be emphasized that freshly isolated LPL contained higher numbers of IL-5-producing cells than did PP. These findings may suggest that more stringent regulation of IgA induction by T cells is required at the site of induction but not at that where IgA synthesis occurs. IL-5-producing CD4+ T_H cells in LPL may need to be present in order for IgA-committed B cells to become IgA producing cells, since IL-5 has been shown to play an important role in IgA synthesis (4).

REGULATION OF HUMAN IgA RESPONSES BY HUMAN IL-6

Since IL-6 is a key cytokine in IgA synthesis, it was important to examine the effect of rhIL-6 on antigen-specific and polyclonal IgA synthesis, including the IgA1 and IgA2 subclasses in humans. When human volunteers were immunized with polysaccharide bacterial vaccines such as the 23-valent pneumococcal carbohydrates by the systemic route, Ag-specific responses were induced predominantly in the IgA isotype (25). Further, when rhIL-6 was added to peripheral blood cell cultures from subjects actively immunized with polyvalent pneumococcal vaccine, in the absence of antigen, Ag-specific IgA synthesis was enhanced. However, the rhIL-6 effect was not isotype-specific, since both IgM and IgG anti-pneumococcal responses were observed. These results also supported the idea that IL-6 is effectively promoting antigen-activated B cells to become high rate Ig-secreting cells.

One of the unique features of the human IgA system is the existence of the IgA1 and IgA2 subclasses, the distribution of which differs in serum and external secretions (26). In serum, approximately 85% of IgA is monomeric IgA1, while external secretions contain more or less equal amounts of polymeric IgA1 and IgA2 antibodies. This varying distribution drew our interest to how rhIL-6 regulates IgA subclass antibody synthesis. When purified human SP B cells from patients with idiopathic thrombocytopenia were incubated with rhIL-6, the number of IgM, IgG, or IgA antibody-producing cells was increased without the addition of mitogen. This result suggested that a subset of SP B cells is naturally activated and can be driven by IL-6 to terminally differentiate. This idea was further investigated by experiments using Percoll density gradient-separated human SP B cells. When Percoll-gradient separated blast B cells were incubated with rhIL-6, higher numbers of mononuclear cells formed IgA-specific spots. However, the small-resting B cells were not affected by rhIL-6. As regards IgA1 and IgA2 synthesis, IL-6 augmented the number of both IgA1 and IgA2 SFC in human SP B cell cultures. Human SP B cells possessed predominantly IgA1-containing cells with less than 20% of IgA2 B cells. Although rhIL-6 enhanced the number of IgA1- and IgA2-producing cells, this cytokine did not alter the ratio of IgA1 to IgA2. Based upon these results, one can suggest that human IL-6 induces activated B cells to terminally differentiate to Ig-producing cells, without any preference for isotype.

SUMMARY

The mucosal immune system provides the major form of immunity in higher mammals, since the majority of lymphoid cells occur in IgA inductive and effector regions, and since the synthesis of IgA represents approximately two-thirds of the total Ig made in humans. Mucosal responses are highly T cell-dependent and recent studies have shown that IL-5 and IL-6 are of most importance in the regulation of IgA synthesis. It is suggested that antigen uptake in GALT results in the induction of $CD4^+$ T_H cells and IgA-committed B cells which, following migration to effector sites such as the lamina propria of intestine, undergo the terminal events resulting in IgA plasma cell formation, IgA synthesis and its transport into external secretions. Thus, activated $CD4^+$ T cells occur in effector sites and the significant proportion of T_H cells which secrete IL-5 (T_{H2}-type) may be responsible for induction of IgA responses in mucosal tissues. In humans, two IgA subclasses, IgA1 and IgA2, occur and the distribution of these subclasses in serum and external secretions is distinct. Our studies suggest that IL-6 is an important cytokine for terminal differentiation to IgA1 and IgA2 synthesis, and thus could be considered as a key mucosal cytokine for local immunity.

ACKNOWLEDGEMENTS

We thank Ms. Amie Stoppelbein for typing this review, Mr. Masahiko Amano for preparation of illustrations and Ms. Kimberly K. McGhee for editorial assistance. Portions of the work described were supported by NIH grants AI 18958, DE 04217, AI 19674, AI 21032, DE 08182, DE 08228, AI 28147, AI 10854, AI 18745 and DK 28537. HK is recipient of RCDA DE 00237.

REFERENCES

1. Mestecky, J., and McGhee, J. R. (1987): *Adv. Immunol.* 40:153-245.
2. Solomon, A. (1980): In: *Cancer Markers*, edited by S. Sell, pp. 57-87, Humana Press, Clifton, NJ.
3. Conley, M. E., and Delacroix, D. L. (1987): *Intern. Med.* 106:892-899.
4. McGhee, J. R., Mestecky, J., Elson, C. O., and Kiyono, H. (1989): *J. Clin. Immunol.* 9:175-199.
5. Heremans, J. F. (1974): In: *The Antigens* Vol. II, edited by M. Sela, p. 365, New York, Academic Press.
6. Bienenstock, J., and Befus, D. (1980): *Immunology* 41:249-261.
7. Butcher, E. C., Rouse, R. V., Coffman, R. L., Nottenburg, C. N., Hardy, R. R., and Weissman, I. L. (1982): *J. Immunol.* 129:2698-2707.
8. Cebra, J. J., Komisar, J. L., and Schweitzer, P. A. (1984): *Annu. Rev. Immunol.* 2:493-548.
9. Craig, S. W., and Cebra, J. J. (1971): *J. Exp. Med.* 134:188-200.
10. Stoolman, L. M. (1989): *Cell* 56:907-910.
11. McGhee, J. R., and Mestecky, J. (1989): *Infect. Dis. Clinics of North America* (in press).
12. Beagley, K. W., Eldridge, J. H., Lee, F., Kiyono, H., Everson, M. P., Koopman, W. J., Hirano, T., Kishimoto, T., and McGhee, J. R. (1989): *J. Exp. Med.* 169:2133-2148.
13. Murray, P. D., McKenzie, D. T., Swain, S. L., and Kagnoff, M. F. (1987): *J. Immunol.* 139:2669-2674.
14. Coffman, R. L., Shrader, B., Carty, J., Mosmann, T. R., and Bond, M. W. (1987): *J. Immunol.* 139:3685-3690.
15. Bond, M. W., Shrader, B., Mosmann, T. R., and Coffman, R. L. (1987): *J. Immunol.* 139:3691-3696.
16. Harriman, G. R., Kunimoto, D. Y., Elliott, J. F., Paetkau, V., and Strober, W. (1988): *J. Immunol.* 140:3033-3039.
17. Lebman, D. A., and Coffman, R. L. (1988): *J. Immunol.* 141:2050-2056.
18. Beagley, K. W., Eldridge, J. H., Kiyono, H., Everson, M. P., Koopman, W. J., Honjo, T., and McGhee, J. R. (1988): *J. Immunol.* 141:2035-2042.
19. Kishimoto, T., and Hirano, T. (1988): *Annu. Rev. Immunol.* 6:485-512.
20. Mosmann, T. R., Cherwinski, H., Bond, M. W., Giedlin, M. A., and Coffman, R. L. (1986): *J. Immunol.* 136:2348-2357.
21. Mosmann, T. R., and Coffman, R. L. (1987): *Immunol. Today* 8:223-227.
22. Coffman, R. L., Seymour, W. P., Lebman, D. A., Hiraki, D. D., Christiansen, J. A., Shrader, B., Cherwinski, H. M., Savelkoul, H. F. J., Finkelman, F. D., Bond, M. W., and Mosmann, T. R. (1988): *Immunol. Rev.* 102:5-28.
23. Taguchi, T., McGhee, J. R., Coffman, R. L., Beagley, K. W., Eldridge, J. H., Takatsu, K., and Kiyono, H. (1990): *J. Immunol. Methods* 128:65-73.
24. Taguchi, T., McGhee, J. R., Coffman, R. L., Beagley, K. W., Eldridge, J. H., Takatsu, K., and Kiyono, H. (1990): *J. Immunol.* (in press).
25. Lue, C., Tarkowski, A., and Mestecky, J. (1988): *J. Immunol.* 140:3793-3800.
26. Mestecky, J., and Russell, M. W. (1986): *Monogr. Allergy* 19:277-301.

Molecular Aspects of Immune Response and Infectious Diseases, edited by H. Kiyono, E. Jirillo, and C. DeSimone. Raven Press, Ltd., New York, © 1990.

9

The Significance of Changes in IgG Carbohydrate in Rheumatoid Arthritis and Tuberculosis

I. M. Roitt*, R. A. Dwek[§], R. B. Parekh[§], T. W. Rademacher[§], C. Warren[§], A. Alavi*, J. S. Axford[+], K. Bodman*, A. Bond*, B. Colaco*, A. Cooke*, P. Delves*, F. C. Hay[+], D. A. Isenberg[+], P. M. Lydyard[+], L. Mackenzie*, G. Rook[‡], M. Smith*, N. Sumar*, and G. Tsoulfa*

Departments of Immunology, [+]Rheumatology Research and [‡]Microbiology, University College and Middlesex School of Medicine, Arthur Stanley House, 40-50 Tottenham Street, [‡]School of Pathology, Riding House Street, London W1P 9PG, U.K.; [§]Glycobiology Unit, Department of Biochemistry, University of Oxford, South Parks Road, Oxford, U.K.

INTRODUCTION

The histological appearance of the joint in rheumatoid arthritis (RA) is consistent with the view that an active immunological process in the deeper layers of the synovium provides a stimulus to the synovial lining cells to grow out as a malign pannus over the surface of the articular cartilage and as a result of the secretion of products of these activated cells, erosion of the cartilage and bone results. It is universally recognized in both seronegative and seropositive adult rheumatoid arthritis, as well as in the various forms of juvenile rheumatoid arthritis, that there is increased reactivity to the patient's own immunoglobulin G (IgG) detected as rheumatoid factors which are known to be present in different major immunoglobulin classes. In particular, IgG rheumatoid factor, being both antigen and antibody within the same molecule, can self-associate to form immune complexes capable of binding IgM rheumatoid factor and complement, thereby activating the acute inflammatory reaction which gives rise to synovial effusions, and contributing to pannus formation through immune complex activation of synovial macrophage-like cells (Figure 1).

77

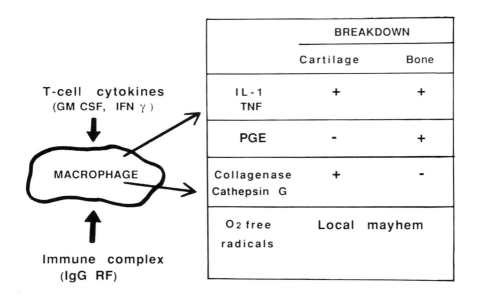

		BREAKDOWN	
		Cartilage	Bone
T-cell cytokines (GM CSF, IFN γ)	IL-1 TNF	+	+
	PGE	-	+
MACROPHAGE	Collagenase Cathepsin G	+	-
Immune complex (IgG RF)	O₂ free radicals	Local mayhem	

FIG. 1. Joint damage due to activated synovial macrophages.

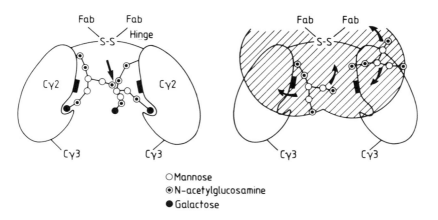

○ Mannose
◉ N-acetylglucosamine
● Galactose

FIG. 2. Left: a schematic representation of an IgG molecule indicating the positions of conserved N-glycosylation sites (at Asn-197 in the Cγ2 domains). The arrow indicates the site of interaction between the α1-3 arms of the two oligosaccharides. The monosaccharide residues of the α1-6 arm of each oligosaccharide are in contact with the surface of the protein. X-ray crystallographic data show a well-defined galactose binding site (3). Unambiguous density information was not obtained for the terminal sialic acid (i.e. Neu5Acα2-6Gal) residue on the α1-6 arm, probably due to the low incidence (<0.1 mole/Cγ2) of this residue. See reference 1. for a list of the oligosaccharide structures present. Right: a schematic representation of an IgG molecule from a patient with rheumatoid arthritis. Note the oligosaccharide chains now terminate with N-acetylglucosamine. The hatched area depicts the possible movement of the oligosaccharide chains.

In view of this central role of IgG autosensitization in the pathogenesis of RA, it is particularly interesting that Parekh et al. (1) were able to demonstrate that the IgG molecules in the serum of patients with RA differed from the normal with respect to the distribution of carbohydrate structures. Human serum IgG is a glycoprotein (1, 2) carrying on average 2.8 N-linked oligosaccharides. Of these, 2.0 are invariably located in the Fc (at the conserved N-glycosylation site of Asn 297), and additional ones in the variable region of the light and heavy chains, with a frequency and position dependent on the occurrence of the N-glycosylation sequon [Asn/Xaa/Ser(Thr)]. Approximately 30 different bi-antennary oligo-saccharides are found to be associated with total human serum IgG and these are distributed non-randomly between the Fab and Fc. The large number of different structures associated with IgG is not the result of studying a polyclonal population, since a similar heterogeneity is found upon analysis of myeloma and hybridoma IgG (2). Characteristics of Fc N-glycosylation include the absence of disialylated structures, a low incidence of monosialylated ones (~10%), and a low incidence of cores with a 'bisecting' N-acetylglucosamine (GlcNAc). Fab N-glycosylation is characterized by a high incidence of di- and monosialylated structures, and of cores with the 'bisecting' GlcNAc residue. Within the Fc, both oligosaccharide-oligosaccharide and oligosaccharide-peptide interactions occur, and these serve to establish the oligosaccharide 'bridge' which holds the two Cγ2 domains apart (Figure 2 left). Of particular significance is the existence of a galactose-binding pocket on each Cγ2 domain, into which the Galβ1 $\rightarrow$ 4 moiety of the α1 $\rightarrow$ 6 arm is able to bind (3).

CARBOHYDRATE ABNORMALITIES IN IgG FROM PATIENTS WITH RHEUMATOID ARTHRITIS

It is now clear that the IgG from patients with rheumatoid arthritis has an increased number of oligosaccharide moieties whose outer arms lack galactose and terminate in N-acetylglucosamine [G(0); Figure 2 right] 'relative' to age-matched normal controls (1, 4). Similar findings with respect to G(0) were also characteristic of patients with juvenile RA further supporting the view that common pathological events may underlie the disease in both its adult and juvenile forms (5).

The galactose defect showed a considerable degree of specificity for RA among the rheumatological disorders. Thus, essentially normal values for G(0) were found for patients with primary SLE, psoriatic arthropathy, ankylosing spondylitis, primary Sjogren's syndrome, myositis, scleroderma and reactive arthritis following infection with yersinia (6). Only in the case of patients with combined SLE and Sjogren's syndrome were elevated G(0) values comparable to those in RA, seen.

It seems likely that the reduction in the number of oligosaccharide chains terminating in galactose can be attributed to a lower activity of the galactose transferase enzyme responsible for addition of galactose residues to terminal N-acetylglucosamine (7). This does not appear to be due to reduced transcription of the galactose transferase activator gene or to be associated with a particular polymorphic form of the gene (unpublished observations with Dr. V. Kidd).

RELATIONSHIP TO PATHOGENESIS

Association between the galactose deficiency and RA does not of course necessarily imply a causative relationship but links with RA under different

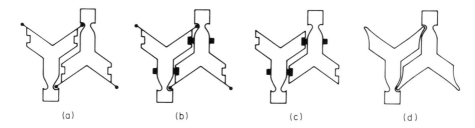

(a)   (b)   (c)   (d)

FIG. 3. A model for the self-association of IgG rheumatoid factors. At least four mechanisms can be envisaged. (a) Insertion of Fab N-linked oligosaccharides (➝) into the vacant carbohydrate-binding site of agalactosyl Fc (see Figure 1). (b) Insertion of Fab N-linked oligosaccharides (➝) into the vacant carbohydrate-binding site of agalactosyl Fc, and binding of the Fab-combining site to a peptide epitope normally covered by the immobile oligosaccharide (see Fig. 1). (c) Binding of the Fab-combining site to a peptide epitope normally covered by the immobile oligosaccharide. (d) Fab peptide image (mimotope) of Fc oligosaccharide binding into the vacant carbohydrate-binding site of agalactosyl Fc.

circumstances are intriguing. Thus, IgG from the MRL/lpr strain of mice which is prone to develop spontaneous arthritis, displays unusually high reactivity with a monoclonal anti-N-acetyl glucosamine (anti-GlcNAc) indicative of a high proportion of oligosaccharide chains lacking galactose. Additionally, the peripheral blood B cells (but curiously not spleen B cells) have a considerably reduced galactosyltransferase activity. In a quite different context, it seems especially relevant that the well-known amelioration of rheumatoid arthritis during pregnancy and the exacerbation which occurs post-partum is paralleled by changes in IgG galactosylation; G(0) drops to very low levels during pregnancy and rises abruptly postnatally.

Defective galactosylation of IgG could contribute to pathogenesis of the disease by facilitating the self-association of IgG rheumatoid factor with a Fab galactose on one molecule binding into the vacant lectin-like pocket in the Cγ2 of another (Figure 3). It is interesting to note that spontaneously aggregated IgG isolated from human plasma shows a selective enrichment of Fab N-linked oligosaccharides. Furthermore, IgG aggregates precipitated from the serum MRL/lpr mice with polyethylene glycol show higher terminal GlcNAc and galactose relative to the monomeric IgG in the supernatant, which could also be consistent with the self-association model.

IS THERE A LINK TO INFECTION?

Examination of IgG galactosylation in the families of patients with RA revealed high G(0) values in 2/8 unrelated spouses. Further studies restricted to the spouses of RA patients showed a similar phenomenon in that 5 out of 20 had G(0) values greater than 2 S.D. above the means of age-related controls. This suggests the operation of an environmental factor, possibly an infectious agent.

We looked at a number of chronic infectious diseases as controls for the galactose defect in RA and although in general, the IgG was normal, tuberculosis provided a dramatic surprise in that G(0) values as high as those seen in RA occurred quite regularly in active disease. The other apparently unrelated disorder in which IgG galactose-deficiency has been observed is Crohn's disease where atypical forms of mycobacteria have been suspected as aetiological agents (8).

Another unexpected finding has been that IgG galactosylation alters following the induction of adjuvant arthritis in rats by complete Freund's adjuvant containing *Mycobacterium tuberculosis* (Warren, 1989 Thesis). The arthritis is effected by T-cells sensitized to a nonapeptide region of the 65kD microbial heat shock protein which cross-reacts with an antigen in the rat joint. It could be significant that Holoshitz et al. (9) showed that T-lymphocytes of RA patients show augmented reactivity to a fraction of mycobacteria cross-reactive with cartilage. In addition, a cross-reaction between mycobacterial and human 65kD heat shock proteins has been demonstrated (Tsoulfa *et al.*, unpublished) at the antibody level and RA patients had considerably enhanced IgG titres to the mycobacterial protein as compared with controls whereas the responses to *E. coli* heat shock proteins was normal.

Numerous strains of mycobacteria and presumably many other microbial species contain proteins with linear sequences which would enable them to cross-react with human proteins at the T-cell level. There is evidence to indicate that whereas a given amino acid sequence within a heterologous protein may both prime and boost auto-reactive T-cells, a similar sequence within the context of a self-protein might only be able to boost already primed cells (Figure 4). One could postulate that appropriate individuals in whom immune responsiveness to the cross-reacting epitope was not adequately controlled could be autosensitized by a microbial stimulus, with the response being perpetuated by the self-epitope. A possible scenario along these lines focused in the joint by human heat shock (stress) proteins in high concentration due to weight bearing or joint activity, could lead to T-cell activation and also to production of agalactosyl IgG and IgG rheumatoid factors which together lead to the joint damage characteristic of the disease (Figure 5).

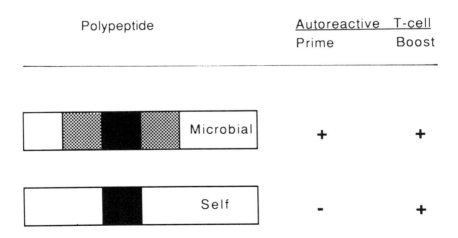

FIG. 4. Stimulation of autoreactive T-cells by cross-reacting linear sequences on microbial protein.

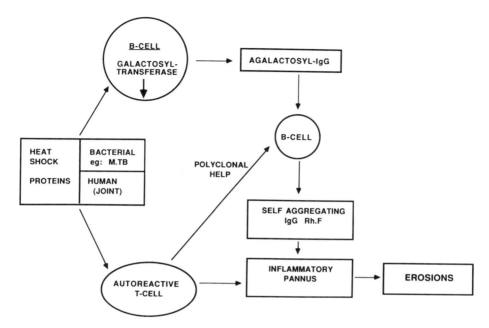

FIG. 5. Hypothesis for role of microbial heat shock proteins in the pathogenesis of rheumatoid arthritis.

REFERENCES

1. Parekh, R. B., Dwek, R. A., Sutton, B. J., Fernandes, D. L., Leung, A., Stanworth, D., Rademacher, T. W., Mizuochi, T., Taniguchi, T., Matsuta, K., Takeuchi, F., Nagano, Y., Miyamoto, T., and Kobata, A. (1985): *Nature* 316:452-457.
2. Rademacher, T. W., Homans, S. W., Parekh, R. B., and Dwek, R. A. (1986): *Biochem. Soc. Symp.* 51:131-148.
3. Sutton, B. J., and Philips, D. C. (1983): *Biochem. Soc. Trans.* 11:130.
4. Parekh, R. B., Isenberg, D. W., Roitt, I. M., Dwek, R. A., and Rademacher, T. W. (1988): *J. Exp. Med.* 167:1731-1736.
5. Parekh, R. B., Ansell, B. M., Isenberg, D. A., Roitt, I. M., Dwek, R. A., and Rademacher, T. W. (1988): *Lancet* i:966-969.
6. Parekh, R. B., Isenberg, D. A., Rook, G., Roitt, I. M., Dwek, R. A., and Rademacher, T. W. (1989): *J. Autoimmunity* 2:101-114.
7. Axford, J. S., Lydyard, P. M., Isenberg, D. A., Mackenzie, L., Hay, F. C., and Roitt, I. M. (1988): *Lancet* ii:1486-1488.
8. Burnham, W. R., Lennard-Jones, J. E., Stanford, J. L., and Bird, R. G. (1978): *Lancet* ii:693-696.
9. Holoshitz, J., Klajman, A., Drucker, I., Lapidot, Z., Yaretzky, A., Frenkel, A., Van Eden, W., and Cohen, I. R. (1986): *Lancet* ii:305-309.

Molecular Aspects of Immune Response and Infectious Diseases, edited by H. Kiyono, E. Jirillo, and C. DeSimone. Raven Press, Ltd., New York, © 1990.

10

Molecular Aspects of Autoimmune Responses to Streptococcal M Proteins

E. H. Beachey*+, G. Majumdar+, M. Tomai*+ and M. Kotb*+

*VA Medical Center, 1030 Jefferson Avenue (151), Memphis, TN 38104 and +University of Tennessee, 956 Court Avenue, Memphis, TN 38163, USA

INTRODUCTION

Infection with group A streptococci may evoke autoimmune diseases in the susceptible host which can affect the heart, kidney, or brain. The major virulence factor of these organisms appears to be the surface antigen, M protein. These are a family of closely-related proteins which emanate from the cell surface as alpha-helical coiled-coil fibrils (1, 2) and define the various serotypes of group A streptococci (3, 4). In the non-immune host, the presence of M protein on the surface of the organisms blocks phagocytosis, whereas in the immune host, type-specific antibodies against the M protein neutralize the anti-phagocytic effect, opsonize the organisms, and render them susceptible to phagocytosis (3). In fact, protective humoral immunity is directed exclusively towards the M protein. However, we and others (5-9) have found that certain serotypes of purified M protein evoke not only protective immune responses, but also autoimmune responses directed against specific host tissue antigens. For these reasons and because of its possible role in the pathogenesis of post-streptococcal sequelae, numerous studies have been dedicated to understanding the nature of the interaction between M protein and the host immune defense mechanisms. The purpose of these studies was not only to develop a safe and effective vaccine against group A streptococcal infections, but also to understand the molecular basis of the autoimmune responses to streptococcal M protein.

Humoral immune responses to M protein have been extensively studied, and several tissue cross-reactive epitopes have been characterized within the primary and/or the quaternary structure of several M protein serotypes (5, 6, 8, 9). The role of antibodies directed toward these cross-reactive determinants in the disease process is not clear, inasmuch as such antibodies have been detected in sera of patients with acute rheumatic fever (10-12) as well as in sera of patients with uncomplicated streptococcal pharyngitis (11). Furthermore, rabbits immunized with various M proteins developed antibodies to several tissue proteins, but had no pathological lesions (6). Thus, it appears that factors other than, or in addition to, autoantibodies are involved in the pathogenesis of the post-infectious sequelae.

Several lines of evidence indicate a possible role of cell-mediated immunity in the pathogenesis of post-streptococcal diseases. The presence of lymphocytic infiltrates in the hearts of acute rheumatic fever patients (13) and of circulating cytotoxic T lymphocytes (CTL) in their blood, which are directed towards cardiac cells (14) strongly suggests a role of T cells in rheumatic carditis. That M protein is involved in these responses has been suggested by several studies, including ours, (15-19) showing that T lymphocytes from all human adults tested respond briskly to purified, pepsin-extracted fragments of M protein (pep M) (18, 19). The response was not merely due to prior exposure to streptococcal infections, inasmuch as cord blood lymphocytes responded in a similar fashion (18). In contrast, T lymphocytes from other species have consistently failed to respond to M protein without prior immunization (18, and our unpublished observation). The unique blastogenic response of human T lymphocytes to M protein is therefore remarkable and suggests the presence of a specific receptor for this antigen on human cells. However, the blastogenic response of human T cells in itself cannot account for the onset of post-streptococcal disease, since it has been estimated that only 10% of the human population are liable to develop disease (20). Functional differentiation of T lymphocytes of some, but not all humans tested can be induced by M protein. Dale and Beachey (19) previously demonstrated that certain serotypes of M protein induce CTL that recognize their targets in an MHC non-restricted manner. Thus, the functional differentiation of T cells induced by M protein may be an important factor in the pathogenesis of these diseases. Clearly, genetic factors, possibly those governed by the MHC genes, control the interaction of M protein with human lymphocytes. The present studies were undertaken to investigate the molecular aspects of the human autoimmune responses to M protein, particularly as they relate to T lymphocytes. We describe data which suggests that M protein acts as a "superantigen," requiring human class II MHC molecules for presentation and a nonpolymorphic receptor on T cells for recognition.

MATERIALS AND METHODS

Purification of M Proteins

M5, M6 and M24 proteins were purified from intact types 5, 6, and 24 groups A streptococci (strains Manfredo, S43, and Vaughan, respectively) by limited pepsin digestion (21). Homogeneity was verified by SDS-polyacrylamide gel electrophoresis (SDS-PAGE). The purified polypeptide fragments are designated pep M5, pep M6, and pep M24.

Cell Preparation

Human peripheral blood mononuclear cells (PBMC) were isolated from freshly prepared buffy coats by Ficoll-Hypaque density gradient centrifugation (22). PB lymphocytes (PBL) were obtained either by using Percoll gradient centrifugation (23) or by collecting the non-adherent cells following an overnight incubation at 37°C and 5% CO_2 in RPMI-1640 medium containing 10% heat-inactivated fetal bovine serum (FBS), glutamine, antibiotic, and antimitotic (RPMI complete medium). Purified T cells were obtained by subjecting PBL to two cycles of E-rosetting using sheep erythrocytes and separating the rosetted cells on a Ficoll-Hypaque gradient (24). E-rosette-positive cells (T lymphocytes) were incubated overnight at 37°C and 5% CO_2 in complete medium to further deplete the adherent cells. E-rosette-negative cells (B lymphocyte-enriched cells) were used as antigen-presenting cells.

Epstein-Barr Virus (EBV) Transformation of B Cells

E-rosette-negative cells were cultured in 96-well U-bottomed plates at various densities (10^3-2 X 10^5 cells per well). Infection with EBV was done by incubating the cells in 100 µl RPMI complete medium containing 5% cell-free B95-8 cell supernatant, which is an EBV-producing cell line. Cultures were fed and monitored for growth. Actively proliferating cells were transferred to 24-well plates and then eventually to culture flasks. EBV-infected B cells were maintained in culture for 3 months and then tested for their ability to present antigen to T lymphocytes.

Analyses of T Lymphocyte Subpopulations

T lymphocyte subpopulations were analyzed with a Coulter EPICS 753 dye-laser flow cytometer with sorting capabilities. All reagents were from Coulter, and the labeling was performed at 4°C. PBL (10^6 cells) were washed once with phosphate-buffered saline (PBS) containing 1 mg/ml bovine serum albumin. The cell pellet was resuspended in 10 µl of phycoerythrin red (PE)-conjugated, anti-CD4 antibody (Coulter) or 10 µl fluorescein (FITC)-conjugated, anti-CD8 antibody (Coulter). To control for nonspecific fluorescence, 10 µl of mouse surface IgG1-FITC plus 10 µl mouse surface IgG1-PE were added to the cell pellet. After 30 min on ice in the dark, the cells were washed 3 times and resuspended in 400 µl PBS plus BSA. In certain experiments, the subpopulations of CD4 subsets [CD4, 4B4 (the helper/inducer population) and the CD4, 2H4 (the suppressor/inducer population)] were also determined by double-labeling (25).

[^{3}H] Thymidine Uptake and Assay of Blastogenic Response

PBL (10^5) were cultured with various concentrations of either pep M5, pep M6, pep M24 or with medium alone in 96-well microtiter plates and incubated at 37°C in a humidified atmosphere of 5% CO_2 for the designated time periods. Four hours before harvesting, the cells were pulsed with 25 µl of 40 µCi/ml [^{3}H] thymidine (sp. act. = 6.7 Ci/mmol, New England Nuclear, Boston, MA), harvested onto glass-fiber paper with an automated cell harvester, and counted in a Packard liquid scintillation counter.

Cytotoxic assays

The target cells used in this study were either Girardi heart cells (GHC), a cell line derived from human myocardium, or K562 erythroleukemia cells, an NK-sensitive target. ^{51}Cr-release microcytotoxicity assays were performed as previously described (19). Briefly, lymphocytes used as effector cells were washed twice in complete RPMI and added to target cells at the ratios indicated in the figure legends. All assays were performed in quadruplicates at 37°C for 3 h after which supernatants were removed using a Skatron supernatant collection system (Skatron, Inc., Sterling, VA) and counted for 1 min each in a gamma counter. Nonspecific ^{51}Cr release was consistently less than 10% of the total for all target cells. Percent specific ^{51}Cr release (percent cytotoxicity) was calculated as follows: [100 x (cpm experimental - nonspecific release) divided by (cpm total - nonspecific release)].

Assay for IL-2 Production

The production of IL-2 by stimulated T cells or T cell lines was determined in a biological assay using a murine IL-2-dependent cell line, CTLL, as described by Gillis *et al.* (26). The CTLL cells were seeded in 96-well plates (10^3-10^4/well) and incubated for 24 h with or without IL-2 containing supernatants or human rIL-2 (Collaborative Research, Boston, MA). Proliferation of CTLL cells was assessed by [^{3}H] thymidine incorporation (3 x 10^4 cpm were equivalent to 1 Unit/ml of activity).

Immobilization of Antigen

Protein antigens were dissolved in Hank's balanced salt solution (HBSS), pH 9.6, added at various concentrations to flat-bottomed 96-well plates, and incubated at 4°C overnight. Before use, the wells were washed twice with RPMI complete. Determination of bound antigen was performed by 1 of 3 procedures: ELISA biotin-avidin assay, or bioassay in which the response of lymphocytes to immobilized antigen is compared to various concentrations of added soluble antigen in the presence of the same number of antigen-presenting cells.

Production of IL-1 and IL-6 Containing Supernatant

PBMC were prepared by Ficoll-Hypaque density gradient centrifugation as described above. 3 x 10^6 cells/ml were cultured overnight at 37°C in 5% CO_2 in RPMI complete medium (20% FBS) containing 1 µg/ml indomethacin. The cell-free supernatants were collected, filter sterilized, and frozen at -20°C and used within two weeks. The IL-1 and IL-6 activities in this supernatant were assessed in bioassays using a T-helper cell line (D10.G4.1) and a murine plasmacytoma cell line, respectively.

T Cell Clones and T Cell Lines

T cell clones were generated by culturing PBMC for 1 week with the appropriate antigen then expanding the responsive cells with 10 U/ml IL-2. Two weeks later some cells were cloned by plating them out in 96-well plates (1-3 cells/well). The remaining cells were maintained in culture with IL-2, irradiated feeder cells and were used in culture as a continuously growing line. T cell clones were intermittently restimulated with antigen and irradiated feeder cells and IL-2. After 7-14 days, proliferating clones were transferred to 24-well plates and eventually to culture flasks. Some T cell clones were screened by flow cytometry to determine the T cell subset phenotype.

The human T cell line, Jurkat, was obtained from Dr. Paul Martin, Seattle, Washington. Another Jurkat line was obtained from Dr. Arthur Weiss or from the American Type Culture Collection (ATCC). HuT-78 and CTLL cells were purchased from ATCC.

RESULTS AND DISCUSSION

Previously we have shown that purified preparations of pep M elicit a strong proliferative response in human PBL (18, 19) composed of by non-adherent CD3+ T cells. The heart cross-reactive serotypes of M proteins (e.g., pep M5, M6, and M19), in addition to stimulating the proliferation of T cells, induced cytotoxic T lymphocytes (CTL) which recognized their targets in an MHC non-restricted manner (19). In contrast, M proteins lacking tissue cross-reactive epitopes (e.g., pep M24) stimulate T cell blastogenesis but do not elicit CTL. Thus, it appears that the primary structure of the M protein molecule plays a role in determining the functional differentiation of the activated human T cells. Studies of the cellular and biochemical changes in human PBL stimulated by these antigens were necessary to understand their role in the pathogenesis of post-streptococcal diseases.

To define the pep M-responding population, phenotypic and functional analyses of T cell subpopulations stimulated with tissue cross-reactive and non-cross-reactive M proteins were performed. PBL were incubated with optimal blastogenic concentrations of either pep M5 or pep M24. The T cell subsets were then analyzed by flow cytometry and tested in functional assays for the presence of cytotoxic or suppressor activity. Cells incubated with pep M5 showed a two-fold increase in the number of CD4,4B4 (helper/inducer) and CD8 (suppressor/cytotoxic) T cells as compared to unstimulated cells (Table 1). The responding populations included CTL as judged by their ability to kill GHC cells (Figure 1). This cytotoxic activity was expressed mainly by CD8 cells, but some activity was also expressed by CD4 cells (19).

Pep M24-stimulated a two-fold increase in the number of CD8 cells but had no effect on the number of CD4,4B4 cells (Table 1). In contrast to pep M5-stimulated cells, pep M24-stimulated cells lacked cytotoxic activity and instead demonstrated suppressor activity which blocked the induction of CTL by either pep M5 or pep M6 (Table 2). The suppressor cells induced by pep M24 did not affect natural killer (NK) activity directed against K562 targets, suggesting that suppression of CTL was specific. Therefore, despite the comparable abilities of the various M proteins to induce human T cell blastogenesis, the responding cells are phenotypically and functionally distinct. Early biochemical events involved in binding, recognition, and signal transduction may account for these differences and could be a function of the primary structure of the M protein molecule itself.

TABLE 1. Stimulation of phenotypically distinct T cell subpopulations
by different serotypes of M protein

Stimulant[a]	Percent of T Cell Subpopulations[b]		
	CD8	CD4,2H4	CD4,4B4
None	15	27	10
	19	25	12
pep M5	30	21	27
	30	ND	27
pep M24	27	22	15
	29	20	13

[a]PBL were cultured for 4 days with medium alone, or with 10 µg/ml of either pep M5 or pep M24. Analysis of T cell subpopulations was done by flow cytometry as mentioned in MATERIALS AND METHODS.
[b]Data from two separate cultures.

An important question is whether M protein is an antigen or a mitogen. Several lines of evidence indicate that M protein is neither a typical antigen nor a typical mitogen. Although M protein stimulates a strong T cell proliferative response, the response has been in most cases lower than the response to PHA. This suggests that a large proportion, but not all T cells, respond to M protein. In addition, we have observed several differences in biochemical reactions triggered in T cells by M protein and PHA (27). However, even if it were a mitogen, it would still be important to determine the basis of its specificity for human T cells in view of its autoimmune properties and the limitation of rheumatic heart disease to the human population.

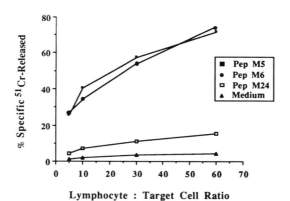

FIG. 1. Induction of cytotoxic T lymphocytes (CTL) by streptococcal M protein. PBL were cultured with RPMI complete medium alone or in the presence of 5 µg/ml pep M5, pep M6, or pep M24. After 5 days, the cells were washed and tested for cytotoxic activity against GHC as described in MATERIALS AND METHODS.

TABLE 2. Induction of suppressor cells by pep M24

| Preincubation[a] | Stimulant | Percent specific [51]Cr Release[b] | |
		GHC	K562
None	Medium	4	35
None	pep M6	32	35
Medium	pep M6	24	26
pep M24	pep M6	6	41

[a]PBL were cultured in medium alone or with 10 µg/ml pep M24. After 3 days in culture, the cells were washed, and 2.5 x 10^4 cells from either culture were mixed with 10^5 fresh autologous cells. These secondary cultures were incubated in medium alone or with 10 µg/ml pep M6.
[b]After 5 days in culture cells were tested for cytotoxicity as described in MATERIALS AND METHODS. The effector : target ration was 100.

Because of the brisk blastogenic response of human T lymphocytes to M protein, we hypothesized that it may bind to these cells via a nonpolymorphic or a relatively invariant receptor. To test our hypothesis, we first studied the response of human T cell clones to M protein. We generated tetanus toxoid (TT) and pep M6-specific T cell clones and tested their ability to respond to TT and pep M6. TT-specific T cell clones responded to both TT and to pep M6, whereas pep M6-specific T cell clones responded to pep M6 but not to TT (Table 3). To exclude the possibility that the response of the TT-specific T cell clones to pep M6 was due to shared epitopes and to provide further evidence for our hypothesis, we tested the response of a human leukemic T cell line (Jurkat), which produces higher levels of IL-2 upon activation. We reasoned that if these CD3[+] Jurkat cells happen to express this nonpolymorphic receptor, they would provide a homogeneous source of T cells.

TABLE 3. Stimulation of human T cell clones with streptococcal M protein[a]

T Cell Clone	Irradiated feeders	Stimulus	[3H]-Thymidine uptake [cpm ± SEM]
T/tt	–	–	507 ± 67
–	+	–	271 ± 73
T/tt	+	–	1,130 ± 321
T/tt	+	TT	13,211 ± 418
T/tt	+	M6	17,188 ± 1134
T/M6	+	TT	298 ± 44
T/M6	+	M6	11,049 ± 44

[a]Cloned 2 x 10^4 T cells specific for either tetanus toxoid (TT) or pep M6 were cultured for 4 days with 10^5 autologous irradiated feeder cells with or without 10 µg/ml of either antigen.

Soluble pep M5 or pep M6 failed to stimulate IL-2 production by Jurkat cells. This was not surprising because of the accessory cell (AC) requirement for the induction of T cell activation by soluble M proteins (see below). Studies by

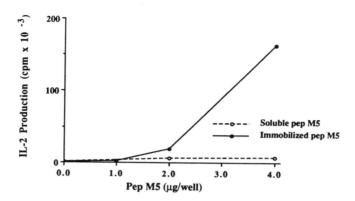

FIG. 2. Production by Jurkat cells stimulated with pep M5. Jurkat cells (10^5/well) were incubated for 24 hrs in 96-well plates with either immobilized or soluble pep M5. The plates were centrifuged, and aliquots of the cell-free supernatant were assayed for IL-2 activity. The method of immobilization of pep M5 and the IL-2 bioassay are described in MATERIALS AND METHODS.

Geppert and Lipsky (28-30) and others (31, 32) showed that in certain AC-dependent T cell responses where the AC are only required to provide a matrix for cross-linking relevant T cell surface molecules, this requirement could be bypassed by immobilizing the antigen on a solid matrix. Based on these reports, we immobilized pep M5 on tissue culture wells and tested its ability to stimulate Jurkat cells added to the wells. Increasing concentrations of immobilized pep M5 induced a marked elevation in IL-2 production by the Jurkat cells, reaching 2.8 U/ml at 4 µg/well, compared to 0.22 U/ml induced by the same or higher concentrations of soluble pep M5 (Figure 2). The ability of immobilized pep M5 to stimulate these leukemic cells depended on the source of the Jurkat cells. In contrast to the Jurkat cells obtained from Dr. John Hansen's laboratory (the results of which are given above), Jurkat cells from Dr. Arthur Weiss' laboratory responded to immobilized pep M5 only in the presence of phorbol ester (PMA) (Table 4). Interestingly, a similar difference in the response of these cells to PMA was reported by the respective laboratories (33, 35). Gillis and co-workers showed direct activation of Jurkat cells by either PMA or PHA alone (33, 34), whereas, Weiss and co-workers clearly demonstrated that the clone of Jurkat cells employed in their laboratory did not produce IL-2 when stimulated by PMA alone (35). Taken together, these observations suggest that immobilized pep M5 by itself is sufficient to activate T cells, provided the necessary machinery is present to transduce the final signal.

In contrast to Jurkat cells, purified human T cells could not be stimulated by immobilized pep M5 alone (Table 5), and the response was only partially reconstituted by PMA (Figure 3). These data suggested that normal purified T cells require yet another signal in addition to that provided by PMA to respond to M protein in the absence of AC. To identify the missing biochemical signal, we tested the ability of known T cell growth factors and cytokines, individually and in combination to reconstitute the proliferative response. Studies by Vine et al. (30) demonstrated that the addition of IL-2 can reconstitute the blastogenic response of purified human T lymphocytes to immobilized PHA. In our system, IL-2 alone or in combination with PMA could not restore the response of purified T cells to

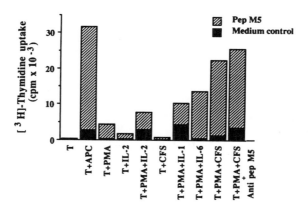

FIG. 3. Reconstitution of T cell response to pep M5 by cytokines. Purified PB T lymphocytes (10^5 cells/well) were incubated for 3 days with or without 10^5 autologous APC. The cells were cultured in either medium alone or with 5 µg/ml pep M5. IL-2 was added at 20 U/ml. IL-1 and IL-6 at 10 U/ml and PMA was at 0.01 µM. The IL-1/IL-6-enriched cell-free supernatant (CFS) was prepared as described in MATERIALS AND METHODS and added at 30 µl/well.

TABLE 4. Signal requirements for the stimulation of two different jurkat cell lines by immobilized pep M5

Cells	Stimulus	IL-2 Production [^{3}H]-Thymidine uptake [cpm ± SEM]
Jurkat[a]	None	1,290 ± 215
	Immobilized pep M5[c]	24,639 ± 6,272
	PMA[d]	8,027 ± 1,149
Jurkat[b]	None	2,869 ± 95
	Immobilized pep M5[c]	3,298 ± 102
	PMA[d]	1,152 ± 70
	PMA + Immobilized pep M5	31,344 ± 1,318

[a]Jurkat cells obtained from Dr. J. Hansen's laboratory.
[b]Jurkat cells obtained from Dr. A. Weiss' laboratory.
[c]Pep M5 was immobilized on the tissue culture wells by adding 40 µg/ml pep M5, incubating for 2 hr and then washing the wells three times.
[d]PMA was added at 0.01 µM.

soluble or cross-linked pep M5. However, total reconstitution was achieved by a combination of cross-linked pep M5, PMA, and an IL-1/IL-6-enriched culture supernatant (Figure 3). The biochemical signals provided by these factors are currently under further investigation.

TABLE 5. Stimulation of purified human T cells with
immobilized pep M5[a]

| Stimulus | [3H]-Thymidine Uptake [cpm ± SEM] | |
	APC Depleted	APC Reconstituted
None	92 ± 20	1,031 ± 158
Soluble pep M5	55 ± 15	22,689 ± 556
Immobilized pep M5	35 ± 8	19,341 ± 2064

[a]T cells (10^5) were purified from PBL by double E-rosetting technique, and then cultured alone or with 10^5 autologous APC (B cell-enriched population). The cells were incubated for 4 days in RPMI complete medium with 5 µg/ml soluble pep M5 or immobilized pep M5 as described in MATERIALS AND METHODS.

Although the above studies support the hypothesis that pep M stimulates T cells via a nonpolymorphic receptor, the nature of this receptor remains to be elucidated. Recently, it has been reported that several bacterial proteins bind to class II molecules and, in turn, bind to relatively invariant regions of the T cell receptor (36-41). These antigens have been designated "superantigens" because of the large population of responding T cells. It has been postulated that because of the polyclonal response, self-reactive T cell clones may be expanded to some threshhold level leading to an autoimmune status (40). Our studies suggest that M protein acts as a superantigen binding to human class II molecules and, in turn, stimulating large populations of T cells.

The superantigens identified thus far have been shown to require MHC class II molecules for presentation, and although there is some MHC restriction, there is no requirement for presentation by syngeneic APC (40-43). We have recently initiated studies of M protein presentation by APC. Antibodies directed to HLA class II antigens, HLA-DR, and DQ inhibited the response of human T lymphocytes to pep

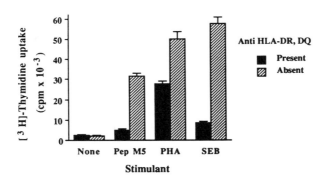

FIG. 4. Inhibition of pep M5-induced blastogenesis by anti-MHC class II antibodies. Purified PB T lymphocytes (10^5 cells/well) were incubated for 3 days with 10^5 irradiated, syngeneic EBV-B cells. PHA, pep M5, and SEB were added at final concentrations of 1%, 5 µg/ml, respectively. Cell-free supernatant containing a monoclonal anti-HLA-DR, DQ was added at 15 µg/well as indicated.

M5 and staphylococcal enterotoxin B (SEB), but had no affect on the response to PHA (Figure 4). In addition, M protein-pulsed EBV-B cells or irradiated normal APC, but not pulsed T cells, resulted in IL-2 production and a blastogenic response (data not shown). Therefore, it appears that class II antigens are required for the M protein response; however, as in the case of SEB and SEA, presentation can be achieved by either syngeneic or allogeneic cells but not by xenogeneic APC (Figure 5). Fixation with paraformaldehyde or treatment with lysomotrophic agents, such as chloroquin, do not affect the ability of APC to present pep M5, PHA, or SEB (data not shown). Our results suggest that processing of M protein may not be required to expose the proper T cell epitope.

The effect of a monoclonal antibody (OKT3) directed against the CD3 component of the T cell receptor also was tested. Anti-CD3 antibody significantly blocked the response of T cells to pep M5 (Figure 6). Moreover, a CD3-mutant of Jurkat cells failed to respond to pep M5 either immobilized or presented by EBV-B cells (data not shown), indicating a possible involvement of the antigen receptor in the response. Although our data suggest that M protein may act as a superantigen, additional studies are ongoing to provide more definitive proof for the binding of M protein to class II antigens and to identify the receptor for M protein on T cells.

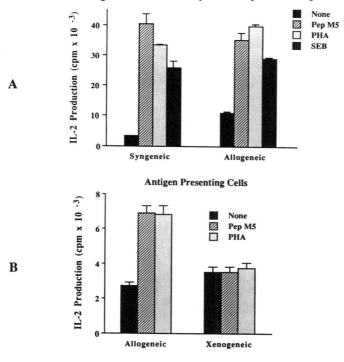

FIG. 5. Presentation of pep M5 by syngeneic, allogeneic, and xenogeneic APC. A) Purified PB T lymphocytes (10^5 cells) were incubated with or without 10^6 irradiated syngeneic or allogeneic APC. B) Jurkat cells (10^5) were incubated for 24 hrs with 10^6 irradiated allogeneic or xenogeneic APC (mouse spleen cells). The cells were stimulated for 24 hrs with either PHA (1%), pep M5 (5 µg/ml), or SEB (10 µg/ml), and aliquots of the cell-free culture supernatant were assayed for IL-2 activity as described in MATERIALS AND METHODS.

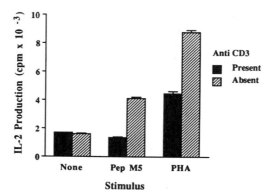

FIG. 6. Inhibition of pep M5-induced IL-2 production by anti-CD3 antibody. CD3+ Jurkat cells (10^5) were incubated with 10^4 irradiated EBV-B cells and stimulated with either PHA (1%) or pep M5 (5 μg/ml) in the presence or absence or anti-CD3 (50 μl of cell-free culture supernatant of an OKT3-producing hybridoma cell line). After 24 hrs in culture, aliquots of the cell-free supernatant were assayed for IL-2 production. There is some nonspecific inhibition by the culture supernatant which was detected using an irrelevant hybridoma. Later experiments were performed using purified OKT3 which inhibited the pep M5 response more significantly.

We have shown that M protein must stimulate T cells via a nonpolymorphic receptor. The response is AC-dependent and requires HLA class II antigens; however, the M protein can be presented to T cells by either syngeneic or allogeneic APC. The requirement for APC can be bypassed by immobilizing M protein, in the case of the Jurkat cells response, or by supplementing the culture with PMA, IL-1, and IL-6, in the case of normal human PB T cells. Our thinking for some time has been that post-streptococcal autoimmune diseases may be the result of molecular mimicry between the M protein and host tissue proteins, and that humoral immunity may be involved in this process. Based on our new findings, our view may need to be modified to envision M protein as a superantigen which may stimulate subsets of T cells with specificity for self-antigens (e.g., cardiac tissue) above a threshold (40) needed to arouse an autoimmune response.

ACKNOWLEDGMENTS

This study was supported by research funds from the U.S. Veterans Administration and by USPHS research grants GM-38530, AI-10085, and AI 13550 to Drs. Kotb and Beachey. The authors wish to thank Ms. Pamela Swann for her excellent secretarial assistance.

REFERENCES

1.   Swanson, J., Hsu, K., and Gotschlich, E. C. (1969): *J. Exp. Med.* 130:1063-1073.
2.   Phillips, G. N., Jr., Flicker, P. F., Cohen, C., Manjula, B. N., and Fischetti, V. A. (1981): *Proc. Natl. Acad. Sci. USA* 78:4689-4693.
3.   Lancefield, R. C. (1962): *J. Immunol.* 89:307-313.

4. Stollerman, G. H. (1975): *Rheumatic Fever and Streptococcal Infection.* Grune and Stratton, New York.
5. Dale, J. B., and Beachey, E. H. (1982): *J. Exp. Med.* 156:1165-1176.
6. Dale, J. B., and Beachey, E. H. (1985): *J. Exp. Med.* 161:113-122.
7. Krisher, K. and Cunningham, M. W. (1985): *Science* 227:413-415.
8. Kraus, W., and Beachey, E. H. (1988): *Proc. Natl. Acad. Sci. USA* 85:4516-4520.
9. Kraus, W., Ohyama, K., Snyder, D. S., and Beachey, E. H. (1989): *J. Exp. Med.* 169:481-492.
10. Kaplan, M. H., and Meyerserian, M. (1962): *Lancet* i:706-710.
11. Kabriskie, J. B., Hsu, K. C., and Seegal, B. C. (1970): *Clin. Exp. Immunol.* 7:147-159.
12. van de Rijn, I., Zabriskie, J. B., and McCarty, M. (1977): *J. Exp. Med.* 146:579-599.
13. Raizada, V., Williams, R., Jr., Chopra, P., and Copinath, N. (1983): *Am. J. Med.* 74:90-96.
14. Hutto, J. H., and Ayoub, E. M. (1980): In: *Streptococcal Diseases and the Immune Response,* edited by S. E. Read and Z. B. Zabriskie, pp. 733-738, Academic Press, New York.
15. Fox, E. N., Wittner, M. K., and Dortman, A. (1966): *J. Exp. Med.* 124:1135-1151.
16. Beachey, E. H., Albert, H., and Stollerman, G. H. (1968): *J. Immunol.* 102:42-52.
17. Beachey, E. H., Seyer, J. H., Dale, J. B., Simpson, W. A., and Kang, A. H. (1981): *Nature* 292:457-459.
18. Dale, J. B., Simpson, W. A., Ofek, I., and Beachey, E. H. (1981): *J. Immunol.* 126:1499-1505.
19. Dale, J. B., and Beachey, E. H. (1987): *J. Exp. Med.* 166:1825-1835.
20. Zabriskie, J. B., and Gibofsky, A. (1986): *Curr. Topics Microbiol. Immunol.* 124:1-20.
21. Beachey, E. H., Stollerman, G. H., Chiang, E. Y., Chiang, T. M., Seyer, J. M., and Kang, A. H. (1977): *J. Exp. Med.* 145:1469-1483.
22. Boyuam, A. C. (1968): *Scand. J. Clin. Lab. Invest.* 21:77-82.
23. Pertoft, H., Rubin, K., Kjellen, L., Laurent, T. C., and Klingeborn, B. (1977): *Exp. Cell Res.* 110:449-457.
24. Kaplan, E., and Clark, C. (1974): *J. Immunol. Methods* 5:131-135.
25. Morimoto, C., Letvin, N.L., Distaso, J. A., Aldrich, W. R., and Scholssman, S. F. (1985): *J. Immunol.* 134:1508-1515.
26. Gillis, S. M., Gorm, M. M., and Smith, K. A. (1978): *J. Immunol.* 120:2027-2032.
27. Kotb, M., and Beachey, E. H. (1989): *Biochem. Biophys. Res. Commun.* 158:803-810.
28. Geppert, T. D., and Lipsky, P. E. (1987): *J. Immunol.* 138:1660-1666.
29. Geppert, T. D., and Lipsky, P. E. (1988): *J. Clin. Invest.* 81:1497-1505.
30. Vine, J. B., Geppert, T. D., and Lipsky, P. E. (1988): *J. Immunol.* 141:2593-2600.
31. Bank, I., and Chess, L. (1985): *J. Exp. Med.* 162:1294-1303.
32. Williams, J. M., Deloria, D., Hansen, J. A., Dinarello, C. A., Loertscher, R., Shapiro, H. M., and Strom, T. B. (1985): *J. Immunol.* 135:2249-2255.
33. Gillis, S., and Watson, J. (1980): *J. Exp. Med.* 152:1709-1719.
34. Dupuis, G., and Bastin, B. (1988): *J. Leukoc. Biol.* 43:238-247.
35. Weiss, A., Wiskocil, R. L., and Stobo, J. D. (1984): *J. Immunol.* 133:123-128.
36. Peavy, D. L., Adler, W. H., and Smith, R. T. (1970): *J. Immunol.* 105:1453-1458.
37. Langford, M. P., Stanton, G. J., and Johnson, H. M. (1978): *Infect. Immun.* 22:62-68.
38. Lynch, D., Cole, B., Bluestone, J., and Hodes, R. (1986): *Eur. J. Immunol.*16:747-751.
39. Kappler, J. W., Staerz, U. D., White, J., and Marrack, P. (1988): *Nature* 332:35-40.
40. White, J., Herman, A., Pullen, A. M., Kubo, R., Kappler, J. W., and Marrack, P. (1989): *Cell* 56:27-35.
41. Mollick, J. A., Cook, R. G., and Rich, R. R. (1989): *Science* 244:817-819.
42. Fleischer, B., Schrezenmeier, H. (1988): *J. Exp. Med.* 167:1697-1707.
43. Janeway, C. A., Jr., Fischer-Lindahl, K., and Hammerling, U. (1988): *Immunol. Today* 9:125-126.
44. Fischer, H., M. Dohlsten, M., Lindvall, M., Sjogren, H. -O., and Carlsson, R. (1989): *J. Immunol.* 142:3151-3157.

Molecular Aspects of Immune Response and Infectious Diseases, edited by H. Kiyono, E. Jirillo, and C. DeSimone. Raven Press, Ltd., New York, © 1990.

11

Antigen Recognition By Class I MHC-Restricted T Cells

J. -C. Cerottini, P. Pala and J. L. Maryanski

Ludwig Institute for Cancer Research, Lausanne Branch, 1066 Epalinges, Switzerland

INTRODUCTION

Antigen recognition by receptors displayed on the plasma membrane of lymphocytes is an essential feature of the immune response. While antigen receptors of B and T cells are well characterized biochemically, the molecular nature of the interaction between antigen and its receptor is still poorly understood. In most T cells, antigen recognition is accomplished by a single heterodimeric structure composed of disulfide-linked α and β chains. Both chains are clonally variable, thus allowing a large diversity of the T cell receptor (TCR) repertoire. Unlike B cells, T cells do not bind intact antigen in solution, but recognize antigen presented in association with products of the major histocompatibility complex (MHC) on the surface of other cells. Among the two major subsets of T cells that express the α/β TCR, CD4+ cells generally recognize antigen in association with class II MHC molecules, whereas CD8+ cells recognize antigen in association with class I MHC molecules. For both CD4+ and CD8+ cells, antigen recognition is clonally restricted to a particular MHC molecule, thus emphasizing the unique specificity of a TCR for a given antigen-MHC combination.

The antigenic moieties recognized in association with class II MHC molecules are usually derived from soluble proteins that have been endocytosed by antigen-presenting cells (APC). There is increasing evidence that presentation of class II-restricted antigen requires endosomal degradation of the foreign protein, followed by intracellular binding of the resulting antigenic peptide fragments to APC class II MHC molecules and transport of the peptide-MHC complexes to the cell surface (these series of events are usually referred to as antigen processing) (1). The major finding in favor of the need for antigen processing in T cell recognition of class II-restricted antigen has been the demonstration that metabolically inactive APC can present proteolytic degradation products or synthetic oligopeptides corresponding

97

to linear segments of antigens, but not intact antigens (2). It is generally assumed that under these conditions, the peptides bind directly to class II MHC molecules at the APC surface, thus bypassing the requirement for intracellular processing. In support of this contention is the demonstration that class II-restricted antigenic peptides bind to soluble class II MHC molecules (3, 4).

In contrast to class II-restricted T cells, class I-restricted CD8$^+$ cells are usually directed against endogenously produced proteins such as viral components, minor histocompatibility antigens and tumor specific transplantation antigens. Until recently, it was assumed that these antigens were integral membrane glycoproteins able to interact with class I MHC molecules at the target cell surface. (As most, if not all, class I-restricted T cells are cytolytic, the readout most often used in these studies is lysis of appropriate target cells expressing the relevant antigen). This assumption was first challenged by the demonstration that viral proteins which were localized in the nucleus of infected cells, such as the large T antigen of SV40 virus (5, 6) and the influenza nucleoprotein (7), could provide target antigens recognized by cytolytic T lymphocytes (CTL). Although the possibility that a few molecules of antigen were present on the target cell plasma membrane could not be ruled out in these initial studies, it is now well established that a class I-restricted antigen does not need to be expressed in its native form at the cell surface to be recognized by T cells. Moreover, there is increasing evidence that the antigenic moieties that are recognized in association with class I MHC molecules are small peptides (presumably resulting from the intracellular degradation of endogenously produced proteins) which are actually bound to the MHC molecules.

In this report, we briefly discuss recent information about recognition of class I-restricted antigens. Since this topic has been reviewed recently (8), we focus primarily on studies performed in our laboratory.

H-2 CLASS I-RESTRICTED RECOGNITION OF THE HLA GLYCOPROTEIN

During the course of a study using mouse tumor cells transfected with genes coding for HLA class I products, we observed that some of the transfectants elicited in syngeneic mice a CTL response that was both HLA-specific and H-2 class I-restricted (9). Thus, from DBA/2 (H-2^d) mice immunized with syngeneic P815 tumor cells transfected with cloned genes coding for HLA-A24 or HLA-CW3, we obtained CTL clones that lysed specifically the corresponding P815-HLA transfectants, but not L cells (H-2^k) transfected with the same HLA genes. However, these clones lysed L cells transfected with both HLA and H-2K^d genes. Similarly, human cells expressing the relevant HLA molecules were not lysed by the CTL clones unless they were transfected with a cloned gene coding for H-2K^d (10). Thus, in this model system, the HLA glycoproteins are recognized as class I-restricted antigens by the murine CTL clones[1].

Footnote 1

It is noteworthy that P815-HLA transfectants can also be used as a source of target cells for human CTL directed against or restricted by the expressed HLA product (11, 12). Therefore, it is evident that different HLA molecular forms are expressed on the surface of the transfectant cells, namely (a) a native form which is integrated in the cell membrane and acts as a class I restriction element and (b) a degraded form, presumably a short peptide, which is bound to the K^d molecule.

Based on the analysis of a large number of independently derived CTL clones, it appears that only K^d, but not D^d or L^d, functions as a class I restriction element in this system. This is consistent with the results of several other studies indicating that single protein antigens can be recognized in association with only certain of the available class I MHC allelic products.

DISSOCIATION BETWEEN SURFACE EXPRESSION OF NATIVE HLA AND CLASS I-RESTRICTED RECOGNITION

Inasmuch as HLA molecules are integral membrane proteins, it was of interest to determine whether expression of the antigen in its native form on the cell surface was required for recognition by class I-restricted CTL clones. To this end, P815 cells which had been transfected with a recombinant gene coding for a secreted form of HLA-CW3 were tested for lysis by the same CTL clones that lysed the P815 transfectants expressing the intact membrane-bound HLA-CW3 molecule. Despite the lack of detectable HLA molecules at the cell surface, the transfectants producing a secreted form of HLA-CW3 were lysed as efficiently as the transfectants expressing large amounts of membrane-associated HLA molecules (13). These results confirmed earlier work with another membrane-associated antigen, the influenza hemagglutinin, which showed that modified forms of the antigen which were not integrated in the plasma membrane were nevertheless recognized efficiently by class I-restricted CTL (14).

As mentioned above, class I-restricted antigens are derived not only from glycoproteins produced on membrane-bound ribosomes but also from proteins synthesized on free ribosomes and destined to the nucleus or the cytosol. It is thus conceivable that cleavage of protein antigens before they are transported to their final destination results in degradation products that are able to bind to class I MHC molecules. According to this hypothesis, it should be possible to express defined class I-restricted antigens in the context of unrelated proteins. Such a possibility was experimentally tested in a recent study using P815 cells transfected with recombinant genes coding for the influenza nucleoprotein in which were inserted synthetic oligonucleotides encoding HLA-CW3 or HLA-A24 amino acid sequences recognized by the anti-HLA CTL clones (15). It was found that P815 cells transfected with nucleoprotein-HLA oligo recombinant genes were lysed efficiently by the anti-HLA CTL clones with a pattern of specificity that corresponded exactly to that obtained on P815 cells transfected with the complete HLA genes. Thus, these experiments, together with other studies using target cells expressing deletion mutants of protein antigens, strongly support the notion that class I-restricted T cells recognize protein degradation products[2].

Footnote 2
Based on the observation that certain class I-restricted antigens can be expressed in cells transfected with subgenic promoterless fragments (16), it has recently been suggested that antigenic peptides are not necessarily protein degradation products, but may be generated directly by transcription and translation of small subgenic regions (17).

SUBSTITUTION OF EXOGENOUS SYNTHETIC PEPTIDES FOR ENDOGENOUSLY-PRODUCED CLASS I-RESTRICTED DETERMINANTS

In a first attempt to identify the antigenic determinants recognized by the anti-HLA-CW3 CTL clones, we used a panel of P815 cells transfected with recombinant exon-shuffled HLA genes. This analysis indicated that the determinants were located within the second external (α2) domain of HLA-CW3 (18). To further define these determinants, we turned to the approach used previously for the identification of class II-restricted determinants, namely the substitution of synthetic peptides for processed antigen. Synthetic peptides corresponding to different linear segments of the HLA-CW3 α2 domain were incubated with normal (HLA$^-$) P815 cells prior to the addition of cloned CTL directed against HLA-CW3. Of the various peptides tested, those corresponding to the C-terminal end of the α2 domain were found to sensitize efficiently target cells for lysis (18, 19). Subsequent experiments established that synthetic peptides corresponding to residues 170-182 of the HLA-CW3 or HLA-A24 provided optimal sensitization of P815 cells for lysis by a series of independently derived CTL clones specific for HLA-CW3 or HLA-A24, respectively (20). It is noteworthy that the 2 HLA alleles differ only at residue 173 within the region 170-182. A clear correlation was found between recognition of P815-HLA transfected cells and recognition of untransfected P815 cells sensitized with HLA peptides. For example, CTL clones that recognized both HLA-CW3 and HLA-A24 transfectants lysed P815 cells in the presence of either peptides, whereas only the corresponding HLA peptide was able to sensitize target cells for lysis by CTL clones that recognized the transfectants mutually exclusively. Moreover, in agreement with the results obtained with transfected cells, it was demonstrated that expression of H-2K^d by target cells was necessary for sensitization by the HLA peptides.

Inasmuch as similar results have been obtained in many different antigenic systems, it is now evident that exogenously added peptides can mimick endogenously produced class I- restricted determinants. Generally, the determinants can be defined with synthetic peptides of 10 to 20 amino acids. The length of the peptide required for optimal sensitization of target cells is usually critical, but varies in different antigenic systems. It should be emphasized that there is no evidence yet that the size of the endogenously produced determinant(s) is identical to the optimal length of the corresponding synthetic peptide. As discussed below, there is suggestive evidence that exogenous antigenic peptides that are recognized by class I-restricted CTL interact with the restricting MHC class I molecules at the target cell surface. Based on the recently defined structure of HLA class I molecules (21), it is thought that the site of interaction is the groove formed by the 2 most external domains of a class I molecule. It is therefore noteworthy that the dimensions of this groove are consistent with the observed length of synthetic peptides recognized by CTL.

COMPETITION BETWEEN PEPTIDES FOR TARGET CELL SENSITIZATION

As discussed before, the two antigenic peptides that mimick the HLA-CW3 or HLA-A24 determinants differ by one amino acid only. If target cell sensitization to CTL-mediated lysis involved binding of these peptides to the same site, it should be possible to demonstrate competition between the peptides for presentation to

CTL. To test this possibility, we took advantage of the availability of CTL clones that recognized the two peptides mutually exclusively. The experiments established that sensitization of target cells by one peptide was drastically inhibited by the addition of the other peptide in excess (20). The inhibition was competitive, since it could be reversed by increasing the concentration of the peptide recognized by the CTL clone used in the assay. Moreover, the competition occurred at the target cell level, as it could be achieved by preincubation of the target cells with both peptides simultaneously, followed by washing, before exposure to CTL.

Based on these results, a series of peptides known to be recognized in association with a given class I or class II MHC molecule were tested for competition using the HLA peptides as reference. While little, if any, competition was observed with the class II-restricted peptides tested, reciprocal competition could be demonstrated between the HLA peptides and another H-2K^d restricted peptide from influenza nucleoprotein (22). A variant form of the nucleoprotein peptide that was known to be 1,000 times more active as an antigen than the natural peptide was found to be at least 30-fold more potent as a competitor. Other peptides from influenza nucleoprotein that are recognized in association with class I MHC molecules other than H-2K^d either failed to compete with the HLA peptides or were only marginally active. Similarly, antigenic peptides from other unrelated antigens which were restricted to H-2D^d or H-2L^d were much less active as competitors as those restricted to H-2K^d, although all 3 class I molecules are well expressed at the surface of P815 cells. Although additional reciprocal competition studies are needed to confirm these findings, it appears likely that the inhibition observed reflects competition between peptides for binding to a single or overlapping sites on a given (e.g. H-2K^d) class I MHC molecule rather than competition for a non-MHC peptide binding protein. Whether exogenous peptides associate directly with class I molecules at the surface of the target cell has yet to be demonstrated, but is suggested by recent studies using glutaraldehyde-fixed target cells or a drug which specifically inhibits transport of newly synthesized class I MHC molecules (23-25).

The general picture that has emerged from in vitro binding studies using peptides and soluble class II MHC molecules is that, although a given class II molecule can bind a variety of unrelated peptides, there is clear selectivity in binding, i.e. a given peptide binds to some class II molecules but not to others (26). This has led to the suggestion that unrelated peptides that bind to the same class II molecule may share a common binding motif (27, 28). In the absence of a reliable assay for binding of peptide to soluble class I MHC molecules, similar studies have not yet been performed in class I-restricted antigenic systems. However, functional competition assays have been used to identify indirectly the residues of a given peptide that are critical for its binding to a class I molecule. For example, analysis of HLA-A24 peptides that had been modified by truncation or by amino acid substitution revealed that 3 residues (Tyr-171, Thr-178 and Leu-179) were critical for the function of the peptide HLA-A24 170-182 as a competitor of H-2K^d restricted peptides (29). As the same 3 residues were present in other competitors, it is conceivable that they constitute an H-2K^d binding motif. Evidence in favor of this contention was provided by the demonstration that a synthetic decapeptide in which a Tyr residue was separated from a Thr-Leu pair by 5 proline residues, with single Ala residues at both ends, competed extremely efficiently with H-2K^d restricted peptides, but not with peptides recognized in association with H-2D^d or H-2L^d. Based on these results, a model for the conformation of the HLA-A24 peptide when bound to the H-2K^d molecule has been proposed (30). While further work is required to confirm the validity of this model, it is likely that the design of functional competitor analogues will facilitate further analysis of the structural properties of peptides that are important for the actual binding to a MHC class I molecule and simplify molecular modelling studies of peptide-class I interactions.

DIVERSITY OF PEPTIDE RECOGNITION BY CTL

In most class I-restricted systems in which the determinants have been identified, there is evidence that the number of distinct immunogenic segments is extremely limited. For example, a limiting dilution analysis of CTL generated in DBA/2 mice immunized with P815-HLA-CW3 transfectants revealed that virtually all the CTL recognized P815 cells sensitized with the peptide HLA-CW3 170-182. As discussed before, these CTL were all H-2K^d restricted. It is noteworthy that region 170-182 is relatively similar between HLA-CW3 and H-2K^d compared to other regions of the molecule (there are 8 residues in common between the mouse and the human 170-182 regions). Hence, it may appear paradoxical that region 170-182 of HLA-CW3, and only this region, is able to provide determinants that elicit CTL responses in DBA/2 mice. This paradox may be reconciled by postulating that this region is the only one in the HLA molecule that contains structural features that allow both binding to K^d and subsequent recognition by some of the TCR available in DBA/2 mice. Alternatively, although there may be other regions in the HLA molecule that have similar structural features, intracellular processing of the antigen may favor the production of peptides derived from region 170-182 over that of other peptides.

The fact that the CTL clones specific for HLA-CW3 all recognize the HLA-CW3 peptide 170-182 does not mean that a single determinant (or epitope) is involved in this antigenic system. Indeed, there is evidence that the clones may differ in their fine specificity. For example, some of the clones recognized exclusively the HLA-CW3 peptide 170-182, whereas other clones clearly crossreacted with the closely related HLA-A24 peptide 170-182, albeit to a varying degree (20). Moreover, 2 clones that recognized exclusively the HLA-CW3 peptide 170-182 on K^d-expressing target cells differed strikingly in their ability to recognize the same peptide presented by target cells expressing a slightly modified K^d molecule (31, 32). It is likely that the differences in fine specificity between CTL clones that recognize the same peptide result from differences in the combining site of their TCR. Such a diversity may reflect differential recognition of a structurally unique peptide MHC-complex. Alternatively, it may be due to the existence of multiple complexes resulting from alternate conformations or orientations of the same peptide within the MHC binding site. Direct binding studies using soluble K^d molecules and peptides, and X-ray crystallographic analysis of peptide-MHC complexes may resolve this issue.

SUMMARY

There is increasing evidence that class I MHC molecules, like class II molecules, bind peptides for presentation to the TCR of CD8$^+$ T cells. The source of these peptides is diverse and includes usually proteins that are synthesized within the presenting cells. As the processing step involved in the production of peptides occurs intracellularly, there is no need for a protein antigen to be expressed in a native form at the surface of the presenting cell. Exogenous synthetic peptides corresponding to linear segments of protein antigens can mimick endogenously-produced class I-restricted determinants. Antigenic peptides from unrelated antigens which are recognized in association with the same class I molecule appear to bind to the same site or to overlapping sites on the restriction molecule. However, identification of the structural features required for binding is still at an early stage. Likewise, very little is known on the various steps involved in antigen processing. The class I-restricted CTL against a given protein antigen are usually directed against very few distinct regions of the molecule, but may be quite diverse in their fine specificity.

REFERENCES

1. Möller, G. (1988): *Immunol. Rev.* 106:5-222.
2. Allen, P. M. (1987): *Immunol. Today* 8:270-273.
3. Babbitt, B. P., Allen, P. M., Matsueda, G., Haber, E., and Unanue, E. R. (1985): *Nature (Lond)* 317:359-361.
4. Buus, S., Colon, S., Smith, C., Freed, J. H., Miles, C., and Grey, H. M. (1986): *Proc. Natl. Acad. Sci. USA* 83:3968-3971.
5. Tevethia, S. S., Tevethia, M. J., Lewis, A. J., Reddy, V. B., and Weissman, S. M. (1983): *Virology* 128:319-330.
6. Gooding, L. R., and O'Connell, K. A. (1983): *J. Immunol.* 131:2580-2586.
7. Townsend, A., McMichael, A. J., Carter, N. P., Huddleston, J. A., and Brownlee, C. G. (1984): *Cell* 39:13-25.
8. Townsend, A., and Bodmer, H. (1989): *Ann. Rev. Immunol.* 7:601-624.
9. Maryanski, J. L., Accolla, R. S., and Jordan, B. R. (1986): *J. Immunol.* 136:4340-4347.
10. Burgert, H. -G., Maryanski, J. L., and Kvist, S. (1987): *Proc. Natl. Acad. Sci. USA* 84:1356-1360.
11. Maryanski, J. L., Moretta, A., Jordan, B., DePlaen, E., Van Pel, A., Boon, T., and Cerottini, J. -C. (1985): *Eur. J. Immunol.* 15:1111-1117.
12. Gomard, E., Begue, B., Sodoyer, S., Maryanski, J. L., Jordan, B. R., and Levy, J. P. (1986): *Nature* 319:153-154.
13. Kahn-Perles, B., Barra, C., Jehan, J., Fourel, D., Barad, M., Maryanski, J. L., and Lemonnier, F. A. (1989): *J. Immunol.* 142:3021-3020.
14. Townsend, A., Bastin, J., Gould, K., and Brownlee, G. G. (1986): *Nature* 324:575-577.
15. Chimini, G., Pala, P., Sire, J., Jordan, B. R., and Maryanski, J. L. (1989): *J. Exp. Med.* 169:297-302.
16. De Plaen, E., Lurquin, C., Van Pel, A., Mariamé, B., Szikora, J. -P., Wölfel, T., Sibille, C., Chomez, P., and Boon, T. (1988): *Proc. Natl. Acad. Sci. USA* 85:2274-2278.
17. Boon, T., and Van Pel, A. (1989): *Immunogenetics* 29:75-79.
18. Maryanski, J. L., Pala, P., Corradin, G., Jordan, B. R., and Cerottini, J. -C. (1986): *Nature (Lond.)* 324:578-579.
19. Pala, P., Corradin, G., Strachan, T., Sodoyer, R., Jordan, B., Cerottini, J. -C., and Maryanski, J. L. (1988): *J. Immunol.* 140:871-877.
20. Maryanski, J. L., Pala, P., Cerottini, J. -C., and Corradin, G. (1988): *J. Exp. Med.* 167:1391-1405.
21. Bjorkman, P. J., Saper, M. A., Samraoui, B., Bennett, W. S., Strominger, J. L., and Wiley, D. C. (1987): *Nature (Lond.)* 329:506-512.
22. Pala, P., Bodmer, H. C., Pemberton, R. M., Cerottini, J. -C., Maryanski, J. L., and Askonas, B. A. (1988): *J. Immunol.* 141:2298-2294.
23. Hosken, N. A., Bevan, M. J., and Carbone, F. R. (1989): *J. Immunol.* 142:1079-1083.

24. Nuchtern, J. G., Bonifacino, J. S., Biddison, W. E., and Klausner, R. D. (1989): *Nature* 339:223-226.
25. Yewdell, J. W., and Bennink, J. R. (1989): *Science* 244:1072-1075.
26. Guillet, J. G., Lai, M. Z., Briner, T. J., Buus, S., Sette, A., Grey, H. M., Smith, J. A., and Gefter, M. L. (1987): *Science (Wash DC)* 235:865-870.
27. Sette, A., Buus, S., Colon, S., Smith, J. A., Miles, C., and Grey, H. M. (1987): *Nature* 328:395-399.
28. Sette, A., Buus, S., Colon, S., Miles, C., and Grey, H. M. (1989): *J. Immunol.* 142:35-40.
29. Maryanski, J. L., Abastado, J. -P., Corradin, G., and Cerottini, J. -C. (1989): *Cold Spring Harbor Symp. Quant. Biol.* (in press).
30. Maryanski, J. L., Verdini, A. S., Weber, P. C., Salemme, F. R., and Corradin, G. (1990): *Cell* (in press).
31. Maryanski, J. L., Abastado, J. -P., and Kourilsky, P. (1987): *Nature (Lond.)* 330:660-662.
32. Maryanski, J. L., Abastado, J. -P., MacDonald, H. R., and Kourilsky, P. (1989): *Eur. J. Immunol.* 19:193-196.

Molecular Aspects of Immune Response and Infectious Diseases, edited by H. Kiyono, E. Jirillo, and C. DeSimone. Raven Press, Ltd., New York, © 1990.

12

Lymphokines and Differential Regulation of T Lymphocyte Responses

F. W. Fitch, T. F. Gajewski, G. Nau, and S. R. Schell

The Committee on Immunology, The Department of Pathology, and the Ben May Institute, University of Chicago, Box 414, 5841 South Maryland Avenue, Chicago, Illinois 60637, USA

INTRODUCTION

Successful recovery from infectious diseases requires an effective immune response in which T lymphocytes have a central role, since they are responsible for cell-mediated immunity and also provide essential "help" for production of humoral antibodies by B lymphocytes. Their participation in immune responses is finely regulated, and subsets of T lymphocytes have distinctive functions which include modulation of the activities of other T cells. The development of cloned normal T cells has greatly facilitated the study of activation requirements and functional characteristics of T cell subsets. Most T lymphocytes can be divided into two subsets, one expressing the CD4 marker and the other expressing CD8. This distinction generally correlates with fundamental functional differences: CD4$^+$ T lymphocytes carry out "helper" function, and their antigen response is restricted by class II MHC molecules. CD8$^+$ T cells are cytotoxic to antigen-bearing target cells and usually are restricted by class I MHC antigens. CD4$^+$ helper T lymphocytes (HTL) appear to exert most of their functions through secreted lymphokines, acting on the T cells that produce them in an autocrine fashion, as well as modulating responses of other cells through paracrine pathways. Stimulated CD8$^+$ cytolytic T lymphocytes (CTL) also secrete some lymphokines, although the array is generally is more restricted, compared to HTL. In addition to having effects on lymphocytes, lymphokines can modulate the activities of cells other than T cells. For example, interferon γ (IFNγ) can activate macrophages for more efficient microbial killing.

Recently, murine CD4$^+$ HTL have been categorized into at least two distinct subsets, designated T_{H1} and T_{H2}, on the basis of the particular array of lymphokines they secrete (1). T_{H1} cells produce IL-2, IFNγ, and lymphotoxin, whereas T_{H2} cells produce IL-4 and IL-5. IL-3 is produced by cells of both subsets, and GM-CSF and tumor necrosis factor are produced preferentially but not exclusively by T_{H1} cells. This distinction also correlates with various functional differences between the cell subsets. IL-2 is the autocrine growth factor for T_{H1} cells which mediate delayed-type hypersensitivity (DTH) (2). IFNγ, produced by T_{H1} cells and CTL but not by T_{H2} cells, activates macrophages (3) and induces increased surface expression of MHC antigens by these cells (4). IL-4 mediates the autocrine growth of T_{H2} cells (5), serves as a cofactor for B cell proliferation (6), enhances IgG1 and IgE production induced by LPS (7), and induces increased surface expression of MHC antigens by B cells (8). Since IL-4 also appears to be required for IgE responses in vivo (9), T_{H2} cells are implicated in allergic reactions. Thus, based on the biological activities of secreted lymphokines, there are two qualitatively different HTL responses, one involving T_{H1} cells, macrophages, and CTL, and the other involving principally T_{H2} cells and B lymphocytes. The characteristics of particular immune responses will be affected significantly by whether T_{H1} or T_{H2} cells predominate.

We have also found that T_{H1} and T_{H2} cells respond differently to several regulatory mechanisms, including some which modulate cell proliferation, and others which affect lymphokine secretion. We will discuss here briefly four regulatory processes, all of them intrinsic to the immune system itself; a more detailed consideration of these issues has been presented elsewhere (10). First, IFNγ inhibits proliferation of T_{H2} but not T_{H1} clones, but lymphokine production by these cells is unaffected. This phenomenon appears to account, at least in part, for the observation that antigen-specific HTL clones are derived in the presence of only IL-2, T_{H2} cells are preferentially obtained while T_{H1} cells are preferentially derived when IFNγ is present in addition to IL-2. Second, T_{H2} cells apparently are stimulated optimally for proliferation by B cells, while optimal proliferation of T_{H1} cells is stimulated by adherent cells, presumably macrophages. However, lymphokine production by both HTL subsets is stimulated by both kinds of antigen-presenting cells (APC). Third, high concentrations of immobilized anti-CD3 mAb dramatically inhibit IL-2-dependent proliferation of T_{H1} cells and CTL, while proliferation of T_{H2} cells in response to IL-2 either is unaffected or is augmented. Fourth, pre-treatment of T_{H1} cells, but not T_{H2} cells or CTL, with IL-2 impairs lymphokine production and proliferation in response to stimulation via the T cell receptor for antigen (TCR); this antigen-unresponsive state appears to involve down-regulation of calcium-dependent signaling. The differential responses of T_{H1} and T_{H2} cells to these several immunoregulatory processes suggests that these mechanisms are major factors which can influence the character of an immune response which develops after antigenic challenge in vivo.

IFNγ INHIBITS PROLIFERATION OF MURINE T_{H2} BUT NOT T_{H1} HTL CLONES

Although IFNγ has a variety of stimulatory activities, including induction of increased expression of MHC antigens (4) and activation of macrophages (3), it also has inhibitory activities including interference with viral replication (11), inhibition of bone marrow cell proliferation (12), and suppression of IL-4-induced B cell proliferation and antibody production (6). We found that anti-IFNγ monoclonal antibody (mAb) overcame the sub-optimal proliferative responses observed when T_{H2} clone D10 cells were stimulated with culture supernatants from T_{H1} clones which contained IFNγ as well as IL-2 or IL-4 (13). This observation suggested that the presence of IFNγ might affect the antigen-induced proliferation of HTL clones since this proliferation is mediated by IL-2 or IL-4. Figure 1

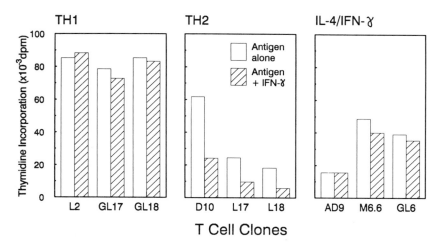

T Cell Clones

FIG. 1. Effect of rIFNγ on proliferation of T_{H1}, T_{H2}, and IL-4/IFNγ clones stimulated with antigen. Cloned T cells (5 x 10^4) were stimulated with 1 x 10^6 syngeneic spleen cells (1000 rad) and OVA (800 μg/ml). IFNγ was added to replicate cultures at a final concentration of 1000 U/ml. ^{3}H-TdR incorporation was measured during the final 6 h of a 48 h incubation. Data are the mean dpm of duplicate cultures, and are representative of at least two experiments.

illustrates the effect of recombinant (r) murine IFNγ on the proliferation of T_{H1} and T_{H2} clones in response to stimulation with antigen; rIL-1 was included in these experiments to obtain maximal proliferation of the T_{H2} clones (14). Proliferation of T_{H2} clones stimulated with antigen was inhibited by rIFNγ, with maximal inhibition generally achieved with 100 U/ml of rIFNγ (data not shown). Proliferation in response to IL-4 or IL-2 also was inhibited, but IL-4-driven proliferation was always inhibited to a greater extent than was IL-2-driven proliferation (13). In contrast, the antigen-induced proliferative response of T_{H1} clones and clones which secrete IL-4 and IFNγ was essentially unaffected by rIFNγ at concentrations up to 1000 U/ml (Figure 1). The response of T_{H1} and IL-4/IFNγ clones to IL-2 also was not affected by rIFNγ (Figure 1). These results suggest that IFNγ inhibits the proliferation of those cells which do not themselves produce IFNγ (T_{H2} cells), but does not affect proliferation of those cells that do (T_{H1} cells and IL-4/IFNγ-producing cells).

However, IL-4 production by T_{H2} clone D10 stimulated by antigen, immobilized anti-CD3 mAb, or the combination of PMA plus ionomycin was unaffected by rIFNγ (13), and similar results have been observed with other T_{H2} clones (data not shown). Therefore, the inhibitory effect of IFNγ appears to be specific for proliferation and is not due to non-specific toxicity. These results also suggest that during the course of an immune response in which IFNγ is present, activated T_{H2} cells could still carry out their lymphokine-mediated effector function even though they might not increase in number.

The selective anti-proliferative effect of IFNγ on T_{H2} but not T_{H1} clones suggested that the type of HTL clone obtained might be influenced if IFNγ were present during derivation of the clones. Therefore, we derived several sets of ovalbumin (OVA)-specific murine HTL clones in the presence of defined concentrations of either rIL-2 alone or rIL-2 in combination with rIFNγ. Data obtained in five independent cloning experiments, indicated that approximately two-thirds of the clones derived in the presence of rIL-2 alone produced IL-4 but not IL-2 and therefore were T_{H2} cells; only 5% of the clones were T_{H1} cells under these conditions. Conversely, approximately two-thirds of the clones derived in the presence of rIL-2 and rIFNγ were T_{H1} cells, with only 6% of the clones being T_{H2} cells (15). Thus, the presence or absence of the single lymphokine, IFNγ, could influence profoundly which HTL subset predominated. A small proportion (5%) of the IL-4-producing clones, and all of the IL-2-producing clones, also produced IFNγ (15).

ADHERENT SPLEEN CELL POPULATIONS STIMULATE PROLIFERATION OF T_{H1} CLONES WHILE SPLENIC B CELLS STIMULATE PROLIFERATION OF T_{H2}

Although antigen processing is required for activation of antigen-specific, class II MHC-restricted, HTL to secrete lymphokines and/or proliferate, many types of cells, including macrophages, B lymphocytes, and Kupffer cells, can carry out this function (16). Synthetic planar lipid membranes containing the relevant class II MHC molecule and a specific peptide which does not require processing can stimulate lymphokine production by T cell hybridomas (17). Thus, the minimal requirement for HTL activation appears to be expression of class II MHC molecules. However, several additional factors seem to be necessary for optimal proliferation of normal HTL clones. Peptide antigen presented by planar membranes not only fails to stimulate proliferation but induces an unresponsive state in T_{H1} clones (18).

When stimulated with whole spleen cells and antigen, both T_{H1} and T_{H2} clones proliferated well, although the magnitude of T_{H2} proliferation often was less than that observed with T_{H1} cells (Figure 2). However, differential responses of T_{H1} and T_{H2} clones were observed when cells were stimulated with antigen and different APC. T_{H1} clones but not T_{H2} clones proliferated optimally when stimulated with antigen and macrophage/dendritic cells enriched by adherence (Figure 2). The poor response of T_{H2} cells was increased only modestly by the addition of IL-1 (data not shown). However when splenic B cells, purified by removal of plastic- and carbonyl iron-adherent cells followed by treatment with anti-Thy-1 plus anti-MAC-1 mAbs and guinea pig complement, were used as APC, T_{H2} but not T_{H1} cells proliferated optimally. The poor response of T_{H1} cells to B cells and antigen was not enhanced by the addition of IL-1 or IL-6 (data not shown). These results indicate that antigen presented by macrophages/dendritic cells preferentially stimulates proliferation of T_{H1} cells while antigen and B cells appear to preferentially stimulate proliferation of T_{H2} clones.

The differential effectiveness of B cells and macrophage/dendritic cells was manifest only when proliferation of T cells was measured; both types of APC stimulated production of equivalent amounts of IL-2 and IL-3 by T_{H1} clones; T_{H2} clones secreted substantial quantities of IL-4 and IL-3 in response to adherent APC, although the amounts were less than that induced by whole spleen or B cell APC (data not shown). Collectively, these results suggest that a poor proliferative response of T_{H1} cells to B lymphocytes and of T_{H2} cells to macrophages is due to the absence of an APC-related component necessary for optimal proliferation but not for lymphokine production. T_{H1} and T_{H2} clones expressed comparable levels of CD3, CD4, and LFA-1, and all of these clones appear to be I-A^k-restricted (data not shown). Thus, the differential effects of macrophages and B cells on the two

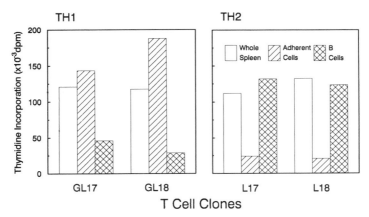

FIG. 2. Proliferation of T_{H1} and T_{H2} clones in response to antigen presented by whole spleen cells, splenic adherent cells, or purified splenic B cells. Cloned T cells (5×10^4) were cultured with 1×10^6 syngeneic spleen cells, 4×10^5 splenic adherent cells, or 1×10^6 purified splenic B cells (1,000 rad) and OVA (800 µg/ml). ^{3}H-TdR incorporation was measured during the final 6 h of a 48 h incubation. Data are the mean dpm of duplicate cultures, and are representative of three experiments.

types of HTL apparently does not involve these structures which have been demonstrated to be involved in interaction of T cells with APC.

Several additional observations support the hypotheses that B cells are the optimal APC for T_{H2} cells and that macrophage/dendritic cells are optimal for T_{H1} activation. The ability of B cells to serve as APC is radiosensitive, whereas antigen presentation by macrophages is unaffected by irradiation (19). Proliferation of T_{H2} clones to whole spleen cells plus OVA was reduced by an average of 60% when the spleen cells were first irradiated with 3,300 R compared to 900 R, while proliferation of T_{H1} cells was unaffected at the higher irradiation dose (data not shown). Also, hepatic non-parenchymal cells, which include Kupffer cells of macrophage/monocyte origin but very few B cells, stimulate optimal proliferation of T_{H1} but not T_{H2} clones (20).

HIGH CONCENTRATIONS OF IMMOBILIZED ANTI-CD3 mAb INHIBIT IL-2-DEPENDENT PROLIFERATION OF T_{H1} AND CTL CLONES BUT NOT T_{H2} CLONES

T cell activation can be achieved using anti-TCR or anti-CD3 mAbs if these mAb are presented in an appropriate array. Immobilized anti-CD3 mAb stimulates lymphokine production by T_{H1}, T_{H2}, and IL-4/IFNγ clones (Figure 3). With each of the HTL clones, increasing concentrations of immobilized anti-CD3 caused production of increasing amounts of lymphokine production (IL-3 and IL-2 or IL-4), and this pattern was observed with all HTL subsets. However, proliferative responses of the various subsets to immobilized anti-CD3 mAb differed considerably (Figure 4). As had been observed previously (21), the dose-response curve for proliferation of T_{H1} clones stimulated with immobilized anti-TCR mAb was biphasic, and IL-2-dependent proliferation of these cells was profoundly inhibited by higher concentrations of immobilized anti-TCR mAb (Figures 4A and

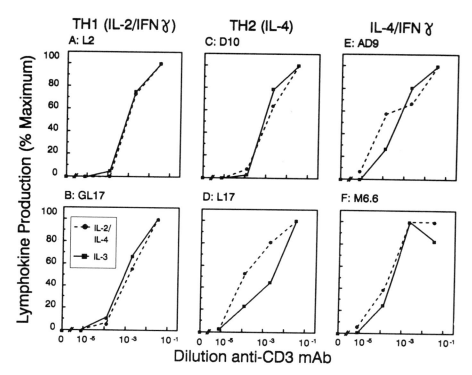

FIG. 3. Lymphokine production by HTL subsets in response to immobilized anti-CD3 mAb. Cloned T cells (5 x 10^4) were cultured with the indicated concentrations of immobilized anti-CD3 mAb (21). After 24 hours, supernatants were collected and analyzed for IL-2 or IL-4 activity and for IL-3 activity. The identity of the T cell growth factor activity, either IL-2 or IL-4, was verified using mAbs 11B11 and S4B6 (15). Lymphokine activities (U/ml) were normalized for comparison. 100% lymphokine production for each of the clones (in U/ml) was: (A) L2: IL-2 = 203, IL-3 = 366,900; (B) GL17: IL-2 = 23, IL-3 = 111,645; (C) D10: IL-4 = 1,120, IL-3 = 17,725; (D) L17: IL-4 = 370, IL-3 = 3,845; (E) AD9: IL-4 = 125, IL-3 = 176,345; (F) M6.6: IL-4 = 230, IL-3 = 23,805. Reprinted with modifications from (10) with permission from Munksgaard.

B). For T$_{H1}$ clones, higher concentrations of immobilized mAb induced greater IL-2 production but were "supraoptimal" for proliferation. This indicates that conditions optimal for lymphokine production by T$_{H1}$ cells are not optimal for proliferation. Optimal proliferation of T$_{H1}$ clones through the autocrine pathway appears to require a precise level of stimulation via the TCR.

In contrast to the inhibitory effect observed with T$_{H1}$ clones, a plateau level of proliferation was typically observed with T$_{H2}$ clones in response to increasing concentrations of immobilized anti-CD3 mAb alone. Anti-CD3 either had no effect or augmented proliferation in response to IL-2 (Figure 4C and D). In addition, anti-CD3 did not affect proliferation of T$_{H2}$ cells stimulated with rIL-4 (data not shown). Thus, T$_{H2}$ clones apparently can secrete lymphokines and proliferate optimally under the same conditions.

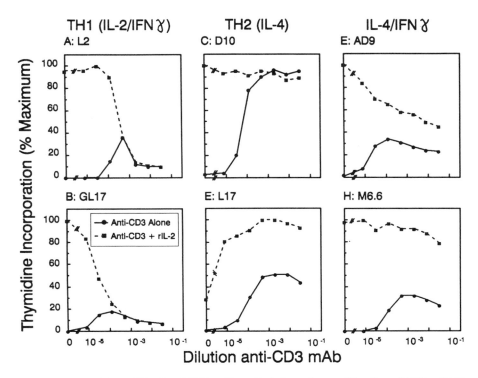

FIG. 4. Effect of immobilized anti-CD3 mAb on IL-2-dependent proliferation of HTL subsets. Cloned T cells (5 x 10^4) were cultured in the presence or absence of rIL-2 (100 U/ml) along with the indicated concentrations of immobilized anti-CD3 mAb (21). ^{3}H-TdR incorporation was assessed for the last 4 hours of the 48 hour incubation. EDTA (0.02 M final concentration) was added to the culture wells 20 min before harvesting to insure removal of adherent cells. Values for mean dpm were normalized for comparison. 100% proliferation (in dpm) for each of the clones was: (A) L2 = 152,550; (B) GL17 = 216,000; (C) D10 = 301,050; (D) L17 = 32,350; (E) AD9 = 322,850; (F) M6.6 = 176,680. Reprinted with modifications from (10) with permission from Munksgaard.

IL-4/IFNγ-producing HTL clones showed a pattern of responsiveness which shared some characteristics of both T$_{H1}$ and T$_{H2}$ proliferation (Figure 4E and F). Similar to the T$_{H2}$ clones, a plateau level of proliferation was typically observed in response to increasing concentrations of immobilized anti-CD3 mAb alone. However, IL-2-dependent proliferation usually was modestly inhibited. Since stimulation with anti-CD3 mAb is thought to mimic stimulation by antigen/MHC, these findings suggest that the concentration of antigen may be important in determining which HTL subset predominates in a particular immunological response. They also suggest that there may be differences between the signaling pathways associated with the TCR or IL-2 receptor in the different T cell subsets.

Stimulation of the TCR is thought to cause hydrolysis of phosphatidyl-inositol 4,5-bisphosphate (PIP$_2$) to yield diacylglycerol and inositol 1,4,5-trisphosphate (IP$_3$) (22). Diacylglycerol presumably activates protein kinase C (PKC), while the IP$_3$ is thought to cause an elevation of intracellular free calcium concentration

($[Ca^{++}]_i$). These signals, in turn, initiate a cascade of biochemical events leading to the eventual transcription of lymphokine genes. This signaling pathway can be mimicked using the pharmacologic agents phorbol myristate acetate (PMA), which activates PKC, and a calcium ionophore that causes a selective influx of calcium ions from the extracellular medium.

We had found previously that PMA and/or ionomycin inhibited IL-2-dependent proliferation effect of high concentrations of immobilized anti-CD3 mAb could be mediated through an elevation of $[Ca^{++}]_i$ and/or PKC activation. Therefore, T_{H1} clones were stimulated with rIL-2 in calcium-free medium and increasing concentrations of immobilized anti-CD3 mAb, with or without added calcium chloride. High concentrations of anti-CD3 only modestly inhibited proliferation of these T_{H1} clones in the absence of calcium; however, proliferation was profoundly inhibited if external calcium was restored (10).

These results suggested that if the anti-proliferative effect of anti-CD3 mAb is mediated through calcium, then either T_{H2} cells do not generate a sufficient calcium increase to inhibit IL-2-dependent proliferation, or they respond differently elevated intracellular calcium. To address this issue, $[Ca^{++}]_i$ levels were measured in T_{H1} and T_{H2} clones following stimulation with Con A, using the calcium indicator dye Indo-1 (24). Although an increase in $[Ca^{++}]_i$ was easily discernable with T_{H1} clones, little or no increase was detectable with T_{H2} clones (10). Calcium increases of 180-500% were observed with T_{H1} clones, but little or no increase (0-11%) was observed with T_{H2} clones (data not shown). Interestingly, resting calcium levels for T_{H2} cells generally were somewhat higher than those of T_{H1} cells. Thus, TCR-associated signaling mechanisms in T_{H1} and T_{H2} clones appear to be different. It is conceivable that different signal transduction mechanisms are linked to distinct biochemical pathways responsible for the eventual expression of subset-specific lymphokine genes.

IL-2-PRETREATMENT INHIBITS RESPONSIVENESS OF T_{H1} CLONES TO ANTIGENIC STIMULATION BUT DOES NOT AFFECT T_{H2} OR CTL CLONES

We have reported previously that HTL clones, but not CTL clones, previously exposed to IL-2 were unresponsive to stimulation by antigen or Con A as reflected by reduced production of lymphokines and failure to proliferate (25, 26). We have found subsequently that this phenomenon is limited to T_{H1} cells. T_{H1} clones, cultured for 48 hours with 100 U/ml rIL-2 and then washed extensively, have impaired proliferative responses when stimulated with immobilized anti-CD3 mAb (Figures 5A and B). However, proliferation of these T_{H1} clones was not affected by pretreatment with 2 U/ml IL-2 or by 1000 U/ml IL-4. Similar results were obtained with several additional T_{H1} clones and following stimulation with antigen or Con A (data not shown). This suboptimal proliferative response was accompanied by a substantial reduction in IL-2 production in response to anti-CD3 mAb, Con A, or antigen (data not shown), suggesting that the reduced level of proliferation resulted from impaired production of the autocrine growth factor for these cells.

In contrast to the results obtained with T_{H1} clones, pretreatment of T_{H2} clones with IL-2 either did not affect or actually resulted in greater proliferation in response to immobilized anti-CD3 mAb. Pretreatment with IL-4 also did not affect subsequent response to immobilized anti-CD3 mAb. Similar results were observed

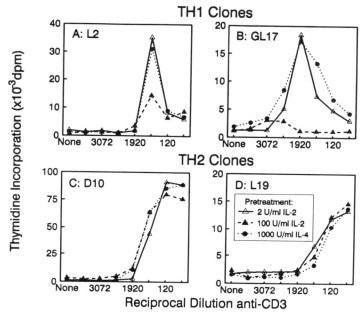

FIG. 5. Effect of pretreatment with IL-2 or IL-4 on subsequent TCR-mediated proliferation of T_{H1} and T_{H2} clones. Cloned T cells (1 x 10^6/ml) were cultured for 2 days with either 2 U/ml or 100 U/ml rIL-2, or 1000 U/ml rIL-4. Cells were then washed extensively, and stimulated with the indicated concentrations of immobilized anti-CD3 mAb. ^{3}H-TdR incorporation was measured during the last 6 h of a 48 h incubation, and results are presented as the mean dpm of triplicate cultures.

when these and several other T_{H2} cells pretreated with IL-2 were stimulated with Con A, or antigen (data not shown). These results implicate a T_{H1}-specific inhibition of TCR signalling events following exposure to IL-2, and again suggest that there are differences in some component of the signalling mechanisms between T_{H1} and T_{H2} cells.

The unresponsive state induced in T_{H1} clones by IL-2 pretreatment apparently involved a defect in calcium-dependent signaling based on two observations. First, elevation of intracellular calcium concentration in response to Con A was reduced in cells pretreated with IL-2 (24, 27). Second, the ability of IL-2-treated cells to produce lymphokines and proliferate in response to antigen was restored upon the addition of a calcium ionophore (26). In addition, recent observations have suggested that the reduced calcium signal in IL-2-pretreated cells correlates with a decrease in the generation of IP$_3$ (27). Thus, exposure of T_{H1} cells to IL-2 causes selective inhibition of calcium-mediated signalling, which appears not to be important for activation of T_{H2}.

REGULATION OF CD8+ CTL PROLIFERATION

All CD8+ CTL clones examined in our laboratory produced IFNγ in response to stimulation through the TCR complex (28, and data not shown). Not surprisingly, the proliferation of these cells in response to IL-2 or antigen was unaffected by IFNγ (data not shown). Our CTL clones did not proliferate in response to IL-4, and their proliferative response was not augmented by IL-1 (data not shown). However, IL-2-dependent proliferation of CTL clones was inhibited by high concentrations of immobilized anti-TCR mAb, even though lymphokine production by these cells approached a maximum at the highest concentration of mAb tested (21). Interestingly, Con A stimulates increased $[Ca^{++}]_i$ in these CTL clones (data not shown). These characteristics suggest some similarities between the activation pathways of CTL and those of T_{H1} cells.

However, regulation of CTL proliferation appears to share two attributes with that of T_{H2} cells. First, proliferation of CTL clones in response to immobilized anti-TCR mAb alone did not show a biphasic dose response curve as did the T_{H1} clones, but rather reached a plateau like the T_{H2} clones (21). This proliferative response appeared to be lymphokine-independent based on the following findings: it was independent of IL-2; CTL proliferation was not transferable by supernatants (29); and these CTL clones did not appear to produce IL-4 (data not shown). Second, pretreatment of CTL clones with IL-2 did not render them unresponsive to subsequent stimulation via the TCR (27). Collectively, these results suggest that CTL signaling pathways have characteristics in common with both T_{H1} and T_{H2} cells.

CONCLUSIONS AND IMPLICATIONS

The segregation of HTL into distinct subsets, which differ in their responses to immunoregulatory processes as well as in the array of secreted lymphokines, has important implications for the control of normal and pathological immune responses. Activation of T_{H1} and T_{H2} cells appears to be antagonistic in several respects, and an improper balance between these two subsets could yield an inappropriate type of immune response. For example, immunity to cutaneous leishmaniasis appears to require the activity of IFNγ, which activates macrophages to kill the protozoal parasite, and therefore depends upon the function of T_{H1} cells and perhaps CTL. T_{H1} cells specific for leishmania antigens have been shown to transfer protection, whereas T_{H2} cells actually appear to exacerbate the disease (30). BALB/c mice are particularly susceptible to this infection, whereas other mouse strains such as C57BL/6 resolve the infection quite readily (30). BALB/c mice may differ in mechanisms controlling T_{H1} or T_{H2} activities.

An understanding of those factors which modulate activation of T_{H1} and T_{H2} cells may facilitate therapeutic intervention. IFNγ appears to be important in the differential regulation of T_{H1} and T_{H2} cells, inhibiting proliferation of T_{H2} but not T_{H1} cells stimulated with exogenous lymphokines or with antigen (15). IFNγ appears to interfere with other effector functions mediated by IL-4, including proliferation of bone marrow cells (12) and Ig production, proliferation, and enhanced class II MHC expression by B cells (7, 8). Preliminary results suggest that T_{H2} cells are obtained more frequently in cultures prepared with primed cells which first have been depleted of CD8$^+$ cells (R. Cron and T. Gajewski, unpublished observations). Thus, activation of IFNγ production may favor an inflammatory-type of cell-mediated immune response, while failure to produce IFNγ would favor production of those antibody isotypes such as IgE and IgA which are dependent on IL-4.

Recent evidence indicates that antigens, such as infectious viruses, which are processed in a cellular compartment other than endosomes, associate preferentially with class I MHC molecules and activate CD8+ CTL effectively. In contrast, other antigens, such as killed virions, bacteria, or soluble protein antigens, which are processed through an endosomal pathway, associate preferentially with class II MHC molecules and activate CD4+ HTL effectively (31). Viral antigens may be processed through both pathways and stimulate both CD8+ CTL and CD4+ HTL. With such antigens, IFNγ secreted by CTL would lead to the preferential activation/differentiation of T_{H2} cells. Extracellular antigens, in the absence of CTL activation, might lead to T_{H2} differentiation.

The putative cellular interactions discussed above are illustrated diagrammatically in Figure 6. Macrophages appear to be the optimal APC for proliferation of T_{H1} cells. Lymphokines produced by activated $T_{H}1$ cells provide a positive feedback for macrophage activation via IFNγ. B cells appear to stimulate optimal proliferation of T_{H2} cells, which, in turn, provide lymphokines that activate B cells. Interactions between the two activation pathways also are evident. IFNγ inhibits several aspects of T_{H2} activation, both at the level of the B lymphocyte and the T cell. Recently, Mosmann and his colleagues have described a factor produced by T_{H2} cells which inhibited the activation of T_{H1} cells but did not affect proliferation in response to mitogens (32). These immunoregulatory pathways provide at least partial explanations for two mutually antagonistic types of immune response, one involving mainly T_{H1} cells and the other mainly T_{H2} cells.

The observation that high concentrations of anti-CD3 mAb inhibit IL-2-dependent proliferation of T_{H1} but not T_{H2} cells suggests that antigen dose may be another important factor which determines the character of the immune response that develops after immunization *in vivo*. DTH without significant antibody production has been observed following immunization with very low doses of antigen, while antibody production occurred following immunization with relatively high antigen concentrations (33). Thus, high doses of antigen might limit the differentiation and expansion of T_{H1} cells, and lead to T_{H2} predominance and, therefore, to antibody production.

There are two important consequences of the antigen-unresponsive state induced by IL-2 in T_{H1} clones: this process serves to limit the duration of the immune response by inhibiting T_{H1} activation and IL-2 production in a negative

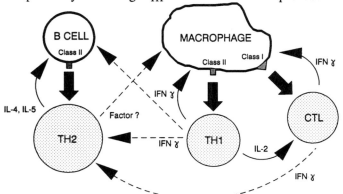

FIG. 6. Summary of postulated regulatory interactions between T_{H1} cells, T_{H2} cells, CTL, B lymphocytes, and macrophages. This diagram is not intended to encompass all functional interactions between the indicated cell types but focuses on those which may be relevant for the differential activation of T_{H1} and T_{H2} cells (see text). Solid lines represent stimulatory signals, whereas dashed lines represent inhibitory signals. Reprinted from (10) with permission from Munksgaard.

feedback fashion, and this feedback also serves to prevent uncontrolled replication of T_{H1} cells by preventing further IL-2 production. Additionally, we have observed that nearly all HTL clones tested to date can effectively lyse antigen-pulsed target cells (data not shown). This mechanism would also limit the duration of the immune response by eliminating APC and thereby interfere with continuing activation of all HTL subsets.

TCR-mediated signalling events also appear to differ between the two cell types. Little or no elevation of intracellular free calcium concentration was observed in T_{H2} cells following stimulation with Con A or anti-CD3 mAb. Expression of subset-specific lymphokine genes may be linked with specific biochemical pathways which are unique to either T_{H1} or T_{H2} cells.

The observations that the several T cell subsets respond differently to high levels of TCR stimulation, to exogenous IFNγ, to pretreatment with IL-2, and to different APC suggest that these are major factors which can influence the character of an immune response which develops after antigenic challenge *in vivo*. Although these mechanisms have not been sufficiently characterized to permit prediction of which T cell subsets will predominate in all situations, it is clear that the various subsets respond differently to these regulatory mechanisms. These differences must be considered when developing strategies for the selective modulation of immune responses.

ACKNOWLEDGEMENTS

This research was supported by grants AI 18061 and CA 44372 from the National Institutes of Health, U.S. Public Health Service. T.F.G. was supported by the Growth and Development Training Grant 2T32 HD-07009 from the U.S. Public Health Service. G.N. was supported by the Medical Scientist Training Program Grant 5T32 GM 07281, and S.R.S. was supported in part by the Lutheran Brotherhood's Medical Research Scholarship. We wish to thank several contributors and collaborators: Genentech, Inc. (South San Francisco, CA), DNAX Research Institute for Molecular and Cellular Biology (Palo Alto, CA), Immunex Corp. (Seattle, WA), and Cetus Corp. (Emeryville, CA) for providing the many recombinant lymphokines and neutralizing mAbs used in these studies; Dr. J. Bluestone (University of Chicago, Chicago, IL) for providing the anti-CD3 mAb; Dr. C. Janeway (Yale University, New Haven, CT) for providing the D10 T_{H2} cell lines; and Dr. D. Magilavy (University of Chicago, Chicago, IL) for providing liver cells used in APC experiments. The expert technical assistance of John Joyce, Peggy Schneider, Michelle Pinnas, Josie Park, and Kris Novak, and the secretarial assistance of Frances Mills, are greatly appreciated.

REFERENCES

1. Mosmann, T.R., and Coffman, R.L. (1989): *Annu. Rev. Immunol.* 7:145-173.
2. Cher, D., and Mosmann, T. (1987): *J. Immunol.* 138:3688-3694.
3. Pace, J., Russell, S., LeBlanc, P., and Murasko, D. (1985): *J. Immunol.* 134:977-981.
4. King, D. P., and Jones, P. P. (1983): *J. Immunol.* 131:315-318.
5. Fernandez-Botran, R., Krammer, P. H., Diamantstein, T., Uhr, J. W., and Vitetta, E. S. (1986): *J. Exp. Med.* 164:580-593.
6. Rabin, E., Mond, J., Ohara, J., and Paul, W. (1986): *J. Immunol.* 137:1573-1576.
7. Coffman, R., and Carty, J. (1986): *J. Immunol.* 136:949-954.

8. Mond, J. J., Carman, J., Sarma, C., Ohara, J., and Finkelman, F. D. (1986): *J. Immunol.* 137:3534-3537.
9. Finkelman, F. D., Katona, I. M., Urban, J. F., Jr., Holmes, J., and Ohara, J. (1988): *J. Immunol.* 141:2335-2341.
10. Gajewski, T. F., Schell, S. R., Nau, G., and Fitch, F. W. (1989): *Immunol. Rev.* 111:79-110.
11. Spitalny, G., and Havell, E. (1984): *J. Exp. Med.* 159:1560-1565.
12. Gajewski, T. F., Goldwasser, E., and Fitch, F. W. (1988): *J. Immunol.* 141:2635-2642.
13. Gajewski, T. F., and Fitch, F. W. (1988): *J. Immunol.* 140:4245-4252.
14. Kaye, J., Gillis, S., Mizel, S. B., Shevach, E. M., Malek, T. R., Dinarello, C. A., Lachman, L. B. and Janeway, C. A., Jr. (1984): *J. Immunol.* 133:1339-1345.
15. Gajewski, T. F., Joyce, J., and Fitch, F. W. (1989): *J. Immunol.* 143:15-22.
16. Grey, H. M., and Chesnut, R. (1985): *Immunol. Today* 6:101-106.
17. Watts, T. H., Brian, A. A., Kappler, J. W. Marrack, P., and McConnell, H. M. (1984): *Proc. Natl. Acad. Sci. (USA)* 81:7564-7568.
18. Quill, H., Gaur, A., and Phipps, R. P. (1989): *J. Immunol.* 142:813-818.
19. Ashwell, J. D., Jenkins, M. K., and Schwartz, R. H. (1988): *J. Immunol.* 141:2536-2544.
20. Magilavy, D. B., Fitch, F. W., and Gajewski, T. F. (1989): *J. Exp. Med.* 170:985-990.
21. Nau, G., Moldwin, R., Lancki, D., Kim, D. -K., and Fitch, F. (1987): *J. Immunol.* 139:114-122.
22. Weiss, A., Imboden, J., Hardy, K., Manger, B., Terhorst, C., and Stobo, J. (1986): *Annu. Rev. Immunol.* 4:593-619.
23. Nau, G. J., Kim, D. -K., and Fitch, F. W. (1988): *J. Immunol.* 141:3557-3563.
24. Otten, G., Herold, K. C., and Fitch, F. W. (1987): *J. Immunol.* 139:1348-1353.
25. Wilde, D. B., Prystowsky, M. B., Ely, J. M., Vogel, S. N., Dialynas, D. P., and Fitch, F. W. (1984): *J. Immunol.* 133:636-641.
26. Otten, G., Wilde, D. B., Prystowsky, M. B., Olshan, J. S., Rabin, L. E. and Fitch, F. W. (1986): *Eur. J. Immunol.* 16:217-225.
27. Schell, S. R., and Fitch, F.W. (1989): *J. Immunol.* 143:1499-1505.
28. Glasebrook, A. L., Kelso, A., Zubler, R. H., Ely, J. M., Prystowsky, M. B., and Fitch, F. W. (1982): In: *Isolation, Characterization and Utilization of T Lymphocyte Clones*, edited by C. G. Fathman and F. W. Fitch, pp. 342-354. Academic Press, New York.
29. Moldwin, R. L., Lancki, D. W., Herold, K. C., and Fitch, F. W. (1986): *J. Exp. Med.* 163:1566-1582.
30. Scott, P., Natovitz, P., Coffman, R. L., Pearce, E., and Sher, A. (1988): *J. Exp. Med.* 168:1675-1684.
31. Braciale, T., Morrison, L., Sweetser, M., Sambrook, J., Gething, M. -J., and Braciale, V. (1987): *Immunol. Rev.* 98:95-113.
32. Mosmann, T. R., Fiorentino, D. E., and Bond, M. W. (1989): *FASEB J.* 3:A1269.
33. Lubet, M.T., and Kettman, J. R. (1978): *Immunogenetics* 6:69-79.

Molecular Aspects of Immune Response and Infectious Diseases, edited by H. Kiyono, E. Jirillo, and C. DeSimone. Raven Press, Ltd., New York, © 1990.

13

The Origin and Nature of Antigen-Binding Factors Having Affinity for Nominal Antigens

K. Ishizaka*, M. Iwata*, H. Ohno*, K. Katamura*,
R. T. Kubo+ and H. M. Grey‡

*The Johns Hopkins University School of Medicine, Baltimore, MD 21239;
+National Jewish Center Immunology & Respiratory Medicine, Denver, CO
80206; and ‡Cytel Corporation, San Diego, CA 92130, USA.*

INTRODUCTION

Antigen specific suppressor T cells (Ts) were described by Gershon and Kondo (1) in 1970. Subsequently, Tada *et al.* (2) confirmed the findings and described that the extracts of suppressor T cells contained a unique factor which has affinity for the nominal antigen, and that this factor could replace the function of Ts. Suppressor T cells and suppressor T cell factor (TsF) were demonstrated in various antigen systems by many investigators and became a fashionable subject in cellular immunology in the next 10 years. After T cell receptors (TCR) were demonstrated, however, many controversial issues were raised on suppressor T cells and suppressor T cell factors. First of all, most suppressor T cell hybridomas could not be stained by anti-CD3, and TCR were not demonstrated on these cells (3). Secondary, suppressor T cells do not have a distinct cell surface marker (4). It was believed that suppressor T cells bear I-J determinant. However, experiments by Uracz *et al.* (5) showed that I-J is not a unique cell surface marker for suppressor T cells. Thirdly, it has been shown that Ts can be enriched by adherence to the wells coated with nominal antigen (6). Indeed, several investigators enriched Ts by this method and constructed T cell hybridomas (7,8). It is well established that T cell receptors on helper and cytotoxic T cells recognize processed antigen in the context of a MHC product, and nominal antigen itself can not stimulate these cells (9). If this principle applies to suppressor T cells, why could nominal antigen bind to suppressor T cells? The same question may be raised to TsF, if the factors are actually a product of T cells. Furthermore, we do not know the mechanisms through which suppressor T cells and/or TsF regulate the antibody response. Nearly 10 years ago, Germain and Benacerraf (10) proposed suppressor T cell network. However, biochemical basis for the network is unknown. In addition to controversial issues on I-J, these problems have to be solved to convince the majority of immunologists for the presence of suppressor T cells and TsF.

When much work on suppressor T cells was going on in 1970-80, we were not involved in this subject. However, we happened to find a TsF-like lymphokine during our studies on the isotype-specific regulation of the IgE antibody response. Furthermore, the antigen-binding lymphokine was quite effective for the regulation of the IgE antibody response. In this article, we would like to discuss some of these controversial issues on TsF and propose possible answers.

NETWORK IN ISOTYPE-SPECIFIC REGULATION OF IgE SYNTHESIS

In the course of our experiments on isotype-specific regulation of the IgE antibody response, we described two T cell factors which have affinity for IgE and selectively regulate the IgE synthesis (11). One of the factors selectively enhances the IgE response, while another factor selectively suppressed the response. The major difference between the IgE-potentiating factors and IgE suppressive factors appears to be carbohydrate moieties in the molecules (12). The IgE-potentiating factors bind to lentil lectin and Con A, while IgE-suppressive factors failed to bind to these lectins. Analysis of cellular mechanisms for the selective formation of either IgE-potentiating factor or IgE-suppressive factors indicated that these factors share a common structural gene and that the carbohydrate moieties in the molecules are decided during the post-translational glycosylation process is controlled by two T cell factors which either enhance or inhibits the process (14). Unique properties of these lymphokines are their biochemical activities. The glycosylation enhancing factor (GEF) appears to be a serine protease, binds to p-amino-benzamidine agarose and could be recovered by elution with benzamidine (15). On the other hand, glycosylation inhibiting factor (GIF) appears to be a derivative of phospholipase inhibitory protein (16). This lymphokine binds to monoclonal antibody against lipomodulin and was recovered by elution at acid pH. The formation of GEF is always accompanied by the formation of IgE-potentiating factor, while the formation of GIF is accompanied by the formation of IgE suppressive factor (17). For example, if one primes BDF1 mice with alum-absorbed ovalbumin for the persistent IgE antibody formation, and stimulates their spleen cells by homologous antigen, the culture supernatant contained both IgE-potentiating factor and glycosylation enhancing factor (GEF), the latter of which had affinity for ovalbumin (18). On the other hand, repeated i.v. injections of OVA into BDF1 mice, which induces the generation of antigen-specific suppressor T cells, facilitates the generation of GIF-producing cells (19). Stimulation of the spleen cells of these mice with OVA results in the formation of IgE-suppressive factors and GIF, which had affinity for OVA. The major cell source of antigen-binding GEF and antigen-binding GIF in these systems were CD4+ (L3T4+) T cells and CD8+ (Lyt 2+) T cells, respectively.

We constructed T cell hybridomas which form GEF or GIF. The representative hybridomas are 12H5 cells and 231F1 cells, respectively. The 12H5 cells constitutively secrete GEF that had no affinity for OVA, but stimulation of these cells with ovalbumin-pulsed H-2b macrophages resulted in the formation of IgE-potentiating factor and OVA-binding GEF (20). Similarly, the 231F1 cells constitutively secrete nonspecific GIF, but stimulation of the cells with OVA-pulsed H-2^d macrophages resulted in the formation of IgE-suppressive factor and OVA-binding GIF (21).

The OVA-binding GEF appears to be similar to antigen-specific augmenting factor previously described by Tokuhisa *et al.* (22). This factor enhances the secondary IgG1 antibody response of DNP-OVA primed spleen cells to homologous antigen in a carrier-specific manner, but could not replace helper T cells (18). The antigen-binding GEF appears to be composed of antigen-binding chain and nonspecific GEF, the latter of which bound to alloantibodies against Ia (20). All of these immunological properties are similar to those of augmenting T cell factor (TaF) (23). On the other hand, OVA-binding GIF from the 231F1 cells suppressed the anti-hapten antibody response of BDF1 mice to DNP-OVA in a carrier-specific manner (21), and appears to be composed of antigen-binding chain and nonspecific GIF which possess I-J determinant (24). Therefore, immunological properties and antigenic structure of OVA-binding GIF are identical to effector type suppressor factors.

ANTIGEN-BINDING FACTORS AND TCR

Cell Sources of OVA-Binding Factors

We examined the presence of TCR on the 12H5 cells and 231F1 cells. The 12H5 cells were well stained by anti-CD3 and anti-TCR$_{\alpha\beta}$, but the 231F1 cells were barely stained by either of the antibodies (Figure 1). Therefore, we enriched the TCR$_{\alpha\beta}^+$ population in the 231F1 cells by repeated cell sorting. After 4 enrichments of TCR$_{\alpha\beta}^+$ cells, we obtained a subclone of 231F1 cells which are well stained by both anti-CD3 (25) and anti-TCR$_{\alpha\beta}$ (26). This clone secreted non-specific GIF, and upon antigenic stimulation with OVA-pulsed syngeneic macrophages, they produced IgE-suppressive factor and OVA-binding GIF. Furthermore, TCR on the 231F1 cells are functional. If one treats the cells with either anti-TCR$_{\alpha\beta}$ or anti-CD3, and the treated cells were incubated in protein A coated wells, these cells formed IgE-binding factor (IgE-BF) and the majority of GIF formed by the cells bound to OVA-Sepharose. Similarly, treatment of the 12H5 cells with either anti-CD3 or anti-TCR$_{\alpha\beta}$ followed by incubation of the treated cells in protein A coated wells resulted in the formation of IgE-BF and OVA-binding GEF. It appears that both the 231F1 cells and 12H5 cells bear functional T cell receptors.

Epitope Specificity of TCR on the Cell Source of Antigen-Binding Factors

Shimonkevitz *et al.* (27) analyzed the epitope in ovalbumin molecules involved in the activation of H-2^d derived OVA-specific T cell hybridomas, and identified a peptide which stimulate the hybridoma cells in the context of Class II molecules. The major immunogenic peptide corresponded to residues 323 to 339 in the original OVA molecule. In collaboration with Dr. Grey, we determined which portion of the OVA molecule is recognized by TCR on the 231F1 cells and 12H5 cells. The 231F1 cells were cultured with H-2^d derived A20.3 cells in the presence of one of the peptides, corresponding to the different portions in the OVA molecules. As shown in Table 1, the cells responded to the peptide 307-317

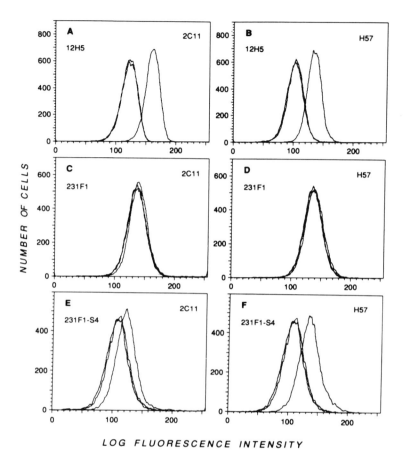

FIG. 1. Cytofluorometric analysis of T cell hybridomas. The cells were stained with either anti-CD3 (145-2C11) or anti-TCR$_{\alpha\beta}$ (H-57) followed by fluoresceinated anti-hamster IgG. 231F1-S4 cells were obtained by enrichment of anti-TCR$_{\alpha\beta}^+$ cells by cell-sorting.

(P307-317) for the formation of IgE-BF but not to the other peptides. It should be noted that antigen-presenting cells are required for stimulation; the peptide itself failed to stimulate the 231F1 cells. The 12H5 cells responded to the same peptide in the presence of the antigen-presenting cells, but not to the other peptides. The response of these hybridoma to the peptide was MHC restricted. The 231F1 cells responded to the peptide for the formation of IgE-BF only when the H-2^d-derived macrophages were employed as antigen-presenting cells. On the other hand, the response of the 12H5 cells was restricted to H-2^b. Furthermore, evidence was obtained that Class II molecules are involved in the antigen presentation. In the experiments shown in Table 2, antigen-presenting cells were fixed with glutaraldehyde and then treated with an appropriate anti-Ia antibody. The hybridoma cells were then cultured with these antigen-presenting cells in the presence of P307-317. The treatment of the A20.3 cells with monoclonal anti-I-A^d

prevented the antigen-presentation to 231F1 cells, while the treatment of I-A^{b+} and I-A^{d+} antigen-presenting cells with anti-IA^b alloantibodies affected the antigen presentation to the 12H5 cells. All of these finding indicate that TCR on the 231F1 cells and 12H5 cells recognize P307-317 in the context of Class II molecules.

TABLE 1. Formation of IgE-BF by stimulation with synthetic peptides[a]

| | T Cell Hybridomas Tested | | | |
| | 231F1 cells | | 125H5 cells | |
Peptide Added	A20.3	% rosette inhibition	LB 27.4	% rosette inhibition
None	+	5 ± 7	+	2 ± 7
111-122	+	1 ± 4	+	4 ± 7
271-285	+	2 ± 1	+	4 ± 7
307-317	+	38 ± 8	+	32 ± 6
307-317	−	4 ± 8	−	3 ± 5
315-325	+	5 ± 7	+	3 ± 6
323-339	+	2 ± 4	+	3 ± 10
370-381	+	2 ± 6	+	4 ± 6
OVA	+	29 ± 7	+	38 ± 9

[a]The 231F1 cells or 12H5 cells were cultured for 24 hr with a peptide in the presence or absence of antigen-presenting cells (A20.3 or LB 27.4) and IgE-binding factors in culture supernatants were detected by rosette inhibition. Because of experimental errors in the percentage of rosette forming cells (RFC), <6% inhibition was not significant.

We wondered that the epitope specificity might be related to the formation of OVA-binding factors. When we constructed T cell hybridomas, in three separate experiments (20,21,28), we have obtained 5 GEF-producing hybridomas and 14 GIF-producing hybridomas. All of these hybridomas produced IgE-binding factors upon incubation with OVA-pulsed syngeneic macrophages, indicating that they are OVA-specific cells. Upon antigenic stimulation, 2 of the 5 GEF producing hybridomas formed OVA-binding GEF, while GEF formed by the other 3 hybridomas failed to bind to OVA-Sepharose. Among the 14 GIF-producing hybridomas, 8 clones produced OVA-binding GIF upon antigenic stimulation. Thus, we stimulated all of the hybridomas with either P307-317 or P323-339 in the presence of syngeneic macrophages. The results shown in Table 3 indicated the correlation between the OVA-binding factor formation and the specificity of TCR. All of the OVA-binding factor-producing hybridomas responded to P307-317 for the formation of IgE-binding factors. On the other hand, all of the other 9 hybridomas, which failed to form OVA-binding factors, failed to respond to this peptide. Indeed, 6 of them responded to P323-339 and formed IgE-BF, but none of them formed OVA-binding factor upon incubation with OVA-pulsed macrophages. The correlation between the epitope specificity of TCR and the formation of OVA-binding factors suggested to us the possibility that the T cell factors may be related to TCR on the cell source of the factors. The amino acid sequence of P307-317 indicate that 7 out of 11 amino acids are hydrophilic (Table 3). The sequence suggests that the peptide may represent a portion of

TABLE 2. Effect of anti-Ia antibodies on the presentation of P307-317 to
T cell hybridomas[a]

T cell hybridomas	Ag-presenting cells	Treatment with	IgE-BF formation (%)[b]
231F1	A20.3	None	46 ± 6
		anti-I-A[d]	0 ± 3
		anti-I-E	41 ± 10
12H5	LB 27.4	None	50 ± 7
		anti-I-A[b]	0 ± 4
		anti-I-A[d]	52 ± 13

[a]Antigen-presenting cells were fixed with glutaraldehyde and then treated with anti-Ia antibodies.
[b]The 231F1 cells or 12H5 cells were co-cultured with fixed antigen-presenting cells, and IgE-binding factors in culture supernatants were assessed by rosette inhibition. The numbers represent the percent of rosette inhibition.

external structure of ovalbumin molecules and therefore that TCR on the OVA-binding factor-forming hybridomas may be specific for the external structure in the antigen molecule.

Specificity of Antigen-Binding Factors

We anticipated that OVA-binding factors from the hybridomas may have affinity for the peptide. To explore this possibility, we stimulated 231F1 cells or 12H5 cells with OVA-pulsed antigen-presenting cells, and OVA-binding factors in the supernatants were partially purified by using OVA-coupled Sepharose. The OVA-binding GIF was then fractionated again on OVA-Sepharose in the presence or absence of a peptide. As shown in Table 4, P307-317 inhibited the binding of the OVA-binding factors to OVA-Sepharose, while P323-339 failed to do so. Similar results were obtained with OVA-binding GEF from the 12H5 cells. The binding of this factor to OVA-Sepharose was inhibited by P307-317. More recently, we coupled the peptide to Sepharose and fractionated the OVA-binding factors. Considering that amino terminus of the peptide may be required for binding to the factors, we obtained the peptide 306-319 and coupled the peptide to Sepharose. As expected, OVA-binding GIF bound to the peptide-coupled Sepharose and were recovered in acid eluates. The same GIF failed to bind to Sepharose coupled with P323-339. The results show that the OVA-binding factors recognize the same epitope as that recognized by TCR on the cell source of the factors. In contrast, the epitope represented by P307-317 is not recognized by anti-OVA antibodies. The binding of ^{125}I-OVA to anti-OVA antibodies was inhibited by unlabeled OVA but not by either P307-317 or P323-339. Thus, OVA-binding factors from 231F1 cells and 12H5 cells bind to a different epitope in OVA-molecules than the majority of anti-OVA antibodies bind.

The common specificity shared by the TCR and antigen-binding factors suggested structural relationship between the two molecules. To study this possibility, we determined as to whether the monoclonal antibodies against TCR

TABLE 3. OVA-binding factor-producing T cell hybridomas respond to
P307-317 for the formation of IgE-BF

Modulators formed	T cell hybridomas	OVA binding factor[a]	IgE-BF formed upon[b]		
			OVA	P307-317[c]	P323-339
GEF	11D5	-	39	4	44
	12H5	+	38	32	3
	21A9	-	35	1	32
	22C2	+	36	33	5
	23A5	-	34	3	34
GIF	231F1	+	36	34	4
	31C2	+	34	31	4
	52A4	+	31	36	4
	52D7	+	30	30	3
	61E7	-	39	3	26
	61E11	-	28	4	30
	62B4	-	37	5	3
	62E10	+	38	32	5
	62F5	-	28	7	9
	64F6	+	31	29	5
	66F3	+	36	32	5
	67B3	-	36	3	5
	71B1	-	37	4	24
	71B4	+	29	34	6

[a]Formation of OVA-binding GEF or OVA-binding GIF, when the hybridoma was stimulated with OVA-pulsed syngeneic macrophages.
[b]The GIF or GEF-producing hybridomas were incubated with syngeneic (BDF1) macrophages in the presence of 10 µg/ml OVA, 2 µg/ml P307-317 or 2 µg/ml P323-339, and IgE-BF in culture supernatants were assessed by rosette inhibition.
[c]S-S-S-A-N-L-S-G-I-S-S.

may bind OVA-binding factors. We purified nonspecific GIF and OVA-binding GIF from 231F1 cells by using anti-lipomodulin Sepharose or OVA-Sepharose, and then fractionated the factors on immunosorbent coated with monoclonal anti-TCR$_{\alpha\beta}$ antibody or anti-TCRα chain from Dr. Ralph Kubo. Nonspecific GIF bound to neither column, but OVA-binding factors bound to both immunosorbent and were recovered by elution at acid pH. Since OVA-binding GIF are composed of antigen-binding chain and nonspecific GIF chain (24), it appears that the antigen-binding chain may not be either α or β chain itself. Ferguson et al. (29,30), obtained monoclonal antibody 14-12 which binds antigen-binding chain of effector suppressor factor (TseF) and another monoclonal antibody 14-30, that binds the antigen-binding chain of inducer type suppressor factor (TsiF). In fact, OVA-binding factor from 231F1 cells was absorbed with 14-12, while OVA-binding factor from the 12H5 cells was absorbed with 14-30. Nonspecific GIF or GEF was not absorbed by either antibody. Thus it appears that the antigen-binding chain of OVA-binding GIF from the 231F1 cells shares the antigenic determinant with TseF, while the antigen-binding chain of 12H5-derived OVA-binding GEF

TABLE 4. Inhibition of the binding of OVA-binding GIF to OVA Sepharose
by a synthetic peptide[a]

Absorption of OVA-GIF in the presence of	GIF activity in OVA Sepharose[b]	
	Effluent	Eluate
PBS	3/41 (−)	42/4 (+)
P307-317	39/6 (+)	15/31 (−)
P323-339	1/41 (−)	38/1 (+)
OVA	31/17 (±)	34/23 (±)
Medium control[c]	0/44	

[a]OVA-binding GIF was fractionated on OVA-Sepharose in the presence or absence of peptide 307-317 or P323-339 or native OVA. After absorption with IgE sepharose, unbound proteins were fractionated on OVA-sepharose. The OVA-Sepharose was eluted with glycine HCl buffer, pH 3.0 to obtain the eluate fractions.
[b]GIF activity in the effluent and eluate fractions was assessed by using the 12H5 cells which produce glycosylated IgE-BF upon incubation with mouse IgE (28). The cells were incubated with IgE in the presence of the effluent or eluate fraction and culture filtrate were fractionated on lentil lectin Sepharose. The numbers in the column represent the distribution of IgE-BF between the effluent/eluate fractions from lentil lectin Sepharose. (+) (−) sign indicate the presence or absence of GIF.
[c]The 12H5 cells were incubated with IgE alone, and IgE-BF in culture filtrate were fractionated on lentil lectin Sepharose, indicating that all IgE-BF was recovered in the eluate fraction.

appears to share a common determinant with TsiF. A question may be raised as to whether the monoclonal antibody may cross-react with a TCR chain. Neither the 14-12 nor 14-30 antibody stained 231F1 or 12H5 cells and neither antibody immunoprecipitated α or β chain on the 12H5 cells. It appears that the antigen-binding chain of the T cell factors possess antigenic determinant, which is lacking in TCR chains. Actual relationship between TCR and antigen-binding factors requires biochemical characterization and gene cloning of the factors. Nevertheless, immunological properties of the factors indicate that the antigen-binding factors are derived from T cells and related to TCR.

POSSIBLE ROLE OF GIF IN Ts CASCADE

In our hypothesis, immunosuppressive effects of antigen-binding GIF is due to GIF chain that has lipomodulin determinant, and represents a derivative of phospholipase inhibitory protein (21). This idea suggested to us the possibility that TsF described by other investigators may have the same biochemical activity. Indeed, collaboration with Dr. Martin Dorf indicated that NP-specific TsF1 and TsF3, derived from their T hybridomas, bound to our anti-lipomodulin Sepharose and were recovered from the column by acid elution (31). The eluate fraction from anti-lipomodulin Sepharose not only suppressed the delayed type hypersensitivity in their systems but also inhibited N-glycosylation of IgE-binding factors in our system. These findings support the hypothesis that the GIF activity or phospholipase inhibitor activity of TsF may play an important role in their immunosuppressive effects. Indeed, our recent experiments indicated that phospholipase A2 inhibitory activity of GIF or TsF may be responsible for the generation of suppressor T cells in the suppressor T cell network.

This series of the experiments were initiated several years ago based on the finding that repeated injections of nonspecific GIF into immunized mice completely suppressed both IgE and IgG antibody responses (32). Spleen cells of the OVA-primed, GIF-treated mice contained OVA-specific suppressor T cells, which could be detected by transfer of the Lyt 2+ T cells into naive mice suggesting that GIF-treatment of antigen-primed mice facilitate the generation of antigen-specific suppressor T cells. Thus, we tried to reproduce this phenomenon in an *in vitro* system. BDF1 mice were primed with alum-absorbed OVA for the persistent IgE antibody response, and their spleen cells obtained 2 weeks after the immunization were stimulated with OVA to activate antigen-primed T cells. The activated T cells were then propagated by IL-2 in the presence or absence of nonspecific GIF. Upon antigenic stimulation with OVA-pulsed syngeneic macrophages, the T cells propagated by IL-2 alone formed IgE-potentiating factor and OVA-binding GEF, while the T cells propagated in the presence of GIF formed IgE-suppressive factor and OVA-binding GIF (33). The cell source of the OVA-binding GIF was Lyt 2+ cells. Thus we constructed T cell hybridomas from the T cells, purified the OVA-binding GIF and assessed for the immunosuppressive effects. As expected, the OVA-binding GIF from the hybridoma suppressed the *in vivo* anti-hapten antibody response to DNP-OVA, but failed to suppress the antibody response to DNP-KLH, indicating that the OVA-binding GIF was antigen-specific TsF (28).

We wondered that phospholipase inhibitory activity of GIF may be responsible for the generation of suppressor T cells. To test this possibility, we determined as to whether well-known phospholipase inhibitors might have the same biologic activities as GIF. We found that recombinant human lipocortin I and synthetic phospholipase A2 (PLA_2) inhibitor, ONO-RS-082, had GIF activity. When the 12H5 cells were cultured with mouse IgE in the presence of a PLA_2 inhibitor, the cells formed unglycosylated IgE-BF, instead of glycosylated IgE-BF. When the 12H5 cells were incubated with IgE alone, essentially all IgE-BF formed by the cells bound to lentil lectin Sepharose. When the same cells were incubated with IgE in the presence of 0.3 nM lipocortin or 0.1 μM ONO-RS-082, essentially all IgE-BF formed by the cells did not have affinity for lentil lectin. In contrast, a well known phospholipase C inhibitor, neomycin, failed to switch the nature of IgE-BF formed by the 12H5 cells. The minimum concentration of lipocortin I and ONO-RS-082 for switching the nature of IgE-BF were comparable to or slightly less than IC 50 of each reagent to inhibit PLA_2, indicating that PLA_2-inhibitory activity of the reagent was responsible for GIF activity (34).

Thus we determined whether the PLA_2 inhibitor might facilitate the generation of suppressor T cells. BDF1 mice were primed with alum-absorbed OVA and their spleen cells were obtained 2 weeks after priming. The antigen-primed T cells were activated by OVA, and the activated T cells were propagated by IL-2 in the presence of a PLA_2 inhibitor or PLC inhibitor. T cells obtained in the cultures were washed, resuspended in fresh culture medium and incubated for 24 hr. As expected, T cells propagated in the presence of lipocortin I or ONO-RS-082 produced GIF, while the same cells propagated in the absence or phospholipase inhibitor or in the presence of neomycin formed GEF. When the same T cells were stimulated with OVA-pulsed syngeneic macrophages, the cells propagated in the presence of either lipocortin or ONO-RS-082 formed IgE-suppressive factors and OVA-binding GIF, while the cells propagated in the presence of neomycin formed IgE-potentiating factors and OVA-binding GEF. The results show that PLA_2 inhibitor facilitated the generation of GIF-producing T cells, and suggest that PLA_2 inhibitory activity of GIF or TsF is responsible for the ability of these lymphokines to generate antigen-specific suppressor T cells (34).

In the suppressor T cell network, Dorf and Benacerraf (35) proposed that TsF1 affected "factor-presenting" macrophages, and facilitates the generation of Ts2, and that TsF2 affect (or modulate) the factor presenting macrophages for the generation of Ts3. However, experimental evidence for this scheme does not exclude the possibility that TsF might directly affect the precursor of suppressor T cells. Since GIF as well as PLA_2 inhibitor could switch the 12H5 cells from the formation of IgE-potentiating factor to the formation of IgE-suppressive factor, we studied the effect of PLA_2 inhibitor on the 12H5 cells. The hybridoma cells were cultured for 3 days in the presence of GIF or 2 μM ONO-RS-082. The cells were recovered and stimulated with OVA-pulsed syngeneic macrophages. The supernatants were appropriately fractionated to determine the nature of IgE-BF formed, and whether the OVA-binding factors formed by the cells had GEF or GIF activity. As shown in Table 5, the 12H5 cells formed OVA-binding GEF upon antigenic stimulation. However, if the hybridoma cells were precultured with GIF of PLA_2 inhibitor, and then stimulated by OVA-pulsed macrophages, the cells formed OVA-binding GIF rather than OVA-binding GEF. Even after fractionation of the factors on p-amino-benzamidine agarose, no GEF activity was detected in the supernatants. As described, the 12H5 cells constitutively form GEF (20). However, after 3 days culture with PLA_2 inhibitor, the cells constitutively secreted GIF rather than GEF. It appears that PLA_2-inhibitor stopped the formation of GEF and induced the formation of GIF. However, the effect of preculture with PLA_2 inhibitor does not appear to last permanently. To test this possibility, the 12H5 cells were cultured for 3 days with PLA_2 inhibitor. The cells were resuspended in fresh culture medium, and cultured for 24, 48 or 72 hr in the absence of PLA_2 inhibitor. The cells were then stimulated with OVA-pulsed syngeneic macrophages. Even after 24 hr in fresh medium, the cells could form OVA-binding GIF. After 72 hr culture in usual medium, however, the same cells formed OVA-binding GEF upon antigenic stimulation.

We wondered that 3 days preculture with PLA_2 inhibitor may not be required for switching the 12H5 cells for the formation of GIF. Thus, we stimulated the 12H5 cells with OVA-pulsed macrophages in the presence of PLA_2 inhibitor and fractionated the OVA-binding factors in the supernatants on anti-lipomodulin Sepharose to determine the presence of GEF or GIF. The results showed that the 12H5 cells formed both the OVA-binding GEF and OVA-binding GIF in the presence of PLA_2 inhibitor. Furthermore, the same results were obtained when the 12H5 cells were pretreated with mitomycin C and then stimulated with OVA-pulsed antigen-presenting cells in the presence of PLA_2 inhibitor. The mitomycin-treated cells formed OVA-binding GIF in the presence of PLA_2 inhibitor. It appears that the same cells had the capacities of making either GEF or GIF under different conditions (36).

A problem to be considered is that the capacity of the 12H5 cells to form GIF may come from BW 5147 which was used to construct the hybridomas. More recently, however, we found that a typical helper T cell clone D10.G4.1 cells could produce GIF in the presence of PLA_2-inhibitor. We found that this T cell clone constitutively secrete GEF and, upon stimulation with conalbumin-pulsed antigen-presenting cells, the T cell clone formed GEF having affinity for conalbumin. Thus, we precultured the D10.G4.1 cells for 3 days with PLA_2 inhibitor ONO-RS-082, together with IL-2. As expected, the cells constitutively secreted GIF. Upon stimulation of the precultured D10.G4 cells with conalbumin-pulsed macrophages, a part of GIF formed by the cells bound to conalbumin. It is not known whether the antigen-binding GIF from the D10.G4 cells has immunosuppressive effects.

TABLE 5. Switching of the 12H5 cells for the formation of GIF by preculture
with phospholipase A$_2$ inhibitor

Experiment	Preculture of 12H5 cells with[a]	OVA MØ	IgE-BF effluent/eluate[b]	OVA-binding factor[c]	
				GEF	GIF
1	None	+	3/34 (IgE-PF)	6/38 (+)	3/43 (-)
	GIF	+	26/9 (IgE-SF)	44/5 (-)	38/6 (+)
	Medium control			47/0	1/40
2	None	+	0/34 (IgE-PF)	0/24 (+)	4/32 (-)
	ONO-RS-082	+	36/2 (IgE-SF)	20/1 (-)	26/1 (+)
	Medium control			34/0	0/25

[a]The 12H5 cells were precultured for 3 days with GIF (Exp. 1) or 2 µM ONO-RS-082 for 3 days. The cells were recovered and stimulated with OVA-MØ.
[b]IgE-BF formed by the cells were fractionated on lentil lectin Sepharose to determine the distribution of the factors between the effluent and eluate fractions.
[c]The supernatants absorbed with IgE-Sepharose were fractionated with OVA-Sepharose to recover OVA-binding factors. Affinity purified OVA-binding factors were fractionated on p-amino-benzamidine agarose. The eluate fractions from the column was assessed for GEF activity, and the effluent fractions were assessed for GIF activity. (+) (-) indicate the presence or absence of GEF/GIF activity.

Nevertheless, the antigen-binding GIF from the D10.G4 cells bound to monoclonal antibody 14-30, which absorb TsiF. Previous work has shown that the cell source of TsiF is L3T4$^+$ T cells. Green *et al.* (37) reported that D10.G4 cells form antigen binding chain of TsiF when they were stimulated with UV-treated, conalbumin-pulsed syngeneic macrophages. These results together with our present findings suggest that some helper T cells may produce inducer type suppressor factor, TsiF, when PLA$_2$ in the cells was inhibited. As described, one of the controversial issues on Ts is that suppressor T cells do not have a unique cell surface marker. Formation of TsiF-like molecules by a typical helper T cell clone suggest that suppressor T cells do not represent a distinct subset of T cells but a phenotype of various T cells which produce GIF under the experimental conditions.

SUMMARY

The cell source of OVA-binding GIF (TsF) or GEF (TaF) appears to express TCR$_{\alpha\beta}$, and respond to anti-CD3 or anti-TCR$_{\alpha\beta}$ for the formation of the factors. The TCR on these cells recognize a unique peptide, corresponding to an external structure of OVA molecules in the context of Class II MHC product, and the OVA-binding factors derived from the cells had affinity for the same epitope. This finding together with cross reaction of the antigen-binding factors with anti-TCR$_{\alpha\beta}$ antibody indicate that the antigen-binding factors are related to TCR.

GIF facilitates the generation of antigen-specific suppressor T cells in antigen-primed T cell populations. This effect is due to PLA$_2$ inhibitory activity of the lymphokine. Evidence was obtained that GIF and PLA$_2$ inhibitor stop the formation of GEF by a T cell hybridoma and a helper T cell clone, and induced the cells to form GIF. The results indicate that the same T cells have the capacities to produce either GIF (TsF) or GEF (TaF) under different conditions, and suggest that the TsF production may not be restricted to a distinct T cell subset.

ACKNOWLEDGEMENTS

This work was supported by research grants AI-11202 and AI-14784 from the U.S.H.H.S.

REFERENCES

1. Gershon, R. K., and Kondo, K. (1970): *Immunology* 18:723-737.
2. Tada, T., Taniguchi, M., and Takemori, T. (1975): *Transplant. Rev.* 26:107-129.
3. Kronenberg, M., Goverman, J., Haars, R., Malissen, M., Kraig, E., Phillips, L., Delvoitch, T., Guciu-Foca, N., and Hood, L. (1985): *Nature* 313:647-653.
4. Moller, G. (1988): *Scand. J. Immunol.* 27:247-250.
5. Uracz, W., Abe, R., and Tada, T. (1985): *Proc. Natl. Acad. Sci. USA* 82:2905-2909.
6. Taniguchi, M., and Miller, J. F. A. P. (1977): *J. Exp. Med.* 146:1450-1454.
7. Weinberger, J., Germain, R. N., Bennacerraf, B., and Dorf, M. E. (1980): *J. Exp. Med.* 152:161-169.
8. Okuda, K., Minami, M., Furusawa, S., and Dorf, M. E. (1981): *J. Exp. Med.* 154:1838-1851.
9. Marrack, P., and Kappler, J. (1986): *Advances in Immunol.* 38:1-30.
10. Germain, R.N., and Benacerraf, B. (1981): *Scand. J. Immunol.* 13:1-10.
11. Ishizaka, K., Suemura, M., Yodoi, J., and Hirashima, M. (1981): *Fed. Proc.* 40:58-62.
12. Yodoi, J., Hirashima, M., and Ishizaka, K. (1982): *J. Immunol.* 128:289-295.
13. Martens, C. L., Jardieu, P., Troustein, M. L., Stuart, S. G., Ishizaka, K., and Moore, K. W. (1987): *Proc. Natl. Acad. Sci. USA* 84:809-813.
14. Ishizaka, K. (1984): *Ann. Rev. Immunol.* 2:159-182.
15. Iwata, M., Munoz, J. J., and Ishizaka, K. (1983): *J. Immunol.* 131:1954-1960.
16. Uede, T., Hirata, F., Hirashima, M., and Ishizaka, K. (1983): *J. Immunol.* 130:878-884.
17. Iwata, M., Huff, T. F., and Ishizaka, K. (1984): *J. Immunol.* 132:1286-1293.
18. Iwata, M., Fukutomi, Y., Hashimoto, T., Sato, Y., Sato, H., and Ishizaka, K. (1987): *J. Immunol.* 138:2561-2567.
19. Jardieu, P., Uede, T., and Ishizaka, K. (1984): *J. Immunol.* 133:3266-3273.
20. Iwata, M., Adachi, M., and Ishizaka, K. (1988): *J. Immunol.* 140:2534-2542.
21. Jardieu, P., Akasaki, M., and Ishizaka, K. (1987): *J. Immunol.* 138:1494-1501.
22. Tokuhisa, T., Taniguchi, M., Okumura, K., and Tada, T. (1978): *J. Immunol.* 120:414-421.
23. Miyatani, S., Hiramatsu, K., Nakajima, P. B., Owen, F. L., and Tada, T. (1983): *Proc. Natl. Acad. Sci. USA* 80:6336-6340.
24. Jardieu, P., and Ishizaka, K. (1987): In: *Immune Regulation by Characterized Polypeptides*, edited by G. Goldstein, F. Bach and H. Witzell, pp. 595-604. Alan R. Liss, Inc., New York.
25. Leo, O., Foo, M., Sacks, D. H., Samuelson, E. E., and Bluestone, J. A. (1987): *Proc. Natl. Acad. Sci. USA* 84:1374-1378.
26. Kubo, R. T., Born, W., Kappler, J. W., Marrack, P., and Pigeon, M. (1989): *J. Immunol.* 142:2736-2742.
27. Shimonkevitz, R., Colon, S., Kappler, J. W., Marrack, P., and Grey, H. M. (1984): *J. Immunol.* 133:2067-2074.
28. Iwata, M., and Ishizaka, K. (1988): *J. Immunol.* 141:3270-3277.
29. Ferguson, T. A., Beaman, K. D., and Iverson, G. M. (1985): *J. Immunol.* 134:3163-3171.
30. Ferguson, T. A., and Iverson, G. M. (1986): *J. Immunol.* 136:2896-2903.

31. Steele, J. K., Kuchroo, V. K., Kawasaki, H., Jaramaman, S., Iwata, M., Ishizaka, K., and Dorf, M. E. (1989): *J. Immunol.* 142:2213-2220.
32. Akasaki, M., Jardieu, P., and Ishizaka, K. (1986): *J. Immunol.* 136:3172-3179.
33. Iwata, M., and Ishizaka, K. (1987): *Proc. Natl. Acad. Sci. USA* 84:2444-2448.
34. Ohno, H., Iwota, M., Nakamura, T., and Ishizaka, K. (1989): *Int. Immunol.* 1:425-433.
35. Dorf, M. E., and Benacerraf, B. (1984): *Ann. Rev. Immunol.* 2:127-157.
36. Ohno, H., Iwata, M., Katamura, K., and Ishizaka, K. (1990): *Int. Immunol.* (in press).
37. Green, D. R., Chue, B., Zhenj, H., Ferguson, T. A., Beaman, K. D., and Flood, P. M. (1987): *J. Mol. Cell. Immunol.* 3:95-108.

Molecular Aspects of Immune Response and Infectious Diseases, edited by H. Kiyono, E. Jirillo, and C. DeSimone. Raven Press, Ltd., New York, © 1990.

14

Antigen Specific MHC Restricted Help Mediated By Cell-Free T Cell Receptor

R. Guy, S. J. Ullrich, M. Foo-Philips, K. S. Hathcock, E. Appella, and R. J. Hodes

Experimental Immunology Branch and Laboratory of Cell Biology, National Cancer Institute, NIH, Bethesda, MD, 20892, USA

INTRODUCTION

The nature of the signals provided to B cells by T_H cells is incompletely understood. One area of controversy involves the question of whether or not, even in conditions of apparently specific T_H cell function, an antigen and MHC-specific effector signal is delivered from T_H cells to B cells. Under certain experimental conditions, the absence of bystander activation of irrelevant B cells suggests a requirement for a specific interaction event between the T_H cell and a B cell in the induction of antibody production by that B cell (1). One interpretation of this finding is that there is a requirement for T_H cells to deliver a specific effector signal directly to those B cells which are activated by that T cell, e.g., via the TCR (2-5). However, an alternative interpretation is that the apparent specificity of T_H-B cell interaction reflects a requirement for intimacy between T_H cell and B cell in the absence of any specific effector signal. Once activated, T_H cells would mediate their helper function by entirely non-specific means, e.g., by the secretion of non-specific lymphokines (6, 7), and the apparent specificity of B cell activation under such circumstances would result from the fact that those B cells which were capable of acting as APC to trigger T_H cells would be closest to the T_H cells at the time of lymphokine release, and would therefore be selectively activated.

In order to further study the mechanism of T_H-dependent (TD) B cell activation, the present study has assessed B cell responses in the absence of T_H cells using supernatants generated by activated cloned T_H cells. These supernatants were capable of replacing T_H cells in hapten specific IgG responses to carrier-hapten conjugate antigens. One essential factor contained in these supernatants was the lymphokine IL-4. In addition, an antigen specific and MHC-restricted factor was identified that could be bound and eluted from monoclonal antibody specific for TCR $V\beta8$ determinants. Thus, antigen specific signals as well as lymphokines generated by the same cloned T_H cells appear to act directly and synergistically in the induction of TD antibody responses.

MATERIALS AND METHODS

Mice

All mice were purchased from The Jackson Laboratory, Bar Harbor, ME.

Antigens

Keyhold limpet hemocyanin (KLH) (Calbiochem-Boehring Corp. American Hoechst Corp. San Diego, CA), fowl gamma globulin (FGG) (N.L. Cappel Laboratories, Cochranville, PA), bovine serum albumin (BSA) (Miles Laboratories, Inc.), and ovalbumin (OVA) (Sigma Chemical Company, St. Louis, MO) were conjugated with 2, 4, 6 trinitrobenzene sulfonate (Pierce Chemical Co., Rockford, IL), as previously described (8).

Immunization

Mice were immunized with 100 µg $TNP^{27}KLH$ or TNP^5OVA in complete Freund's adjuvant (Difco Laboratories, Detroit, MI) intraperitoneally 1-12 months before use.

Culture Medium

Medium used was RPMI 1640 supplemented with 100U/ml penicillin, 100 µg/ml streptomycin, 10 mM hepes, 0.1 mM nonessential amino acids, 1 mM sodium pyruvate, 2 mM L-glutamine, $5 \times 10^{-5}M$ 2-mercaptoethanol, and 10% fetal calf serum (FCS).

Clones

T cell clones used in this study were previously described (9-11).

Reagents

Monoclonal anti-CD3ε antibody 145-2C11 was kindly provided by Dr. J.A. Bluestone (12). The anti-IL-4 mAb 11B11 was kindly provided by Dr. W.E. Paul and Dr. J. Ohara (13). Anti-IL-2 mAb S4B6 was a gift from Dr. T. Mosmann (14). Anti-Thy-1 mAb was a kind gift from Dr. P. Lake (15). Anti-TCR Vβ8 monoclonal antibody F23.1 was prepared from cells generously provided by Dr. M. Bevan (Scripps Research Foundation, La Jolla, CA) (16). Murine recombinant IL-4 (rIL-4) (Immunex Corp., Seattle, WA) was generously provided by Dr. W.E. Paul (17). Human rIL-2 was a generous gift from Cetus Corp. (Emeryville, CA).

Preparation of T_H Supernatant

Clone supernatants were derived either by stimulation with specific antigen or by stimulation with immobilized anti-CD3 antibody as previously described (18).

In Vitro Antibody Production

TNP-KLH primed T depleted spleen cells were cultured with either T helper cells or with T clone supernatant in the presence or absence of 0.01 or 0.001 µg/ml TNP-KLH or TNP-FGG. On day 4 of culture, medium was removed and replaced with fresh medium containing no antigen (18). Supernatant samples were collected between days 7 and 14 of culture for assay of antibody production.

Assays of Antibody Response

Antibody responses were assayed either as:

A. Plaque forming cells (PFC) responses were measured on day 5 of culture by assaying on TNP-conjugated sheep erythrocytes (TNP-SRBC) as previously described (19).

B. Enzyme-linked immunosorbent assays (ELISA) of TNP-binding antibody were carried out as previously described (20). The amount of TNP-specific antibody measured in these assays is reported as optical density (O.D.) or as µg/ml of anti-TNP antibody based on a standard curve that was generated using affinity-purified mouse anti-TNP antibody.

Absorption and Elution of Antigen-Specific Helper Factor (ASHF)

Supernatants were incubated with Sepharose 4B beads conjugated with F23.1 (anti-TCR Vβ8 antibody), bovine serum albumin, or monoclonal antibody specific for Ly6 as previously described (21). Supernatants from these absorptions were then assayed for helper activity. Adsorbed material was eluted from Sepharose beads by treatment with 0.01M acetic acid followed by neutralization. The resulting material was assayed for helper activity in the presence of added rIL-2 (50 U/ml) and rIL-4 (100 U/ml).

RESULTS

Activated T_H Clone Supernatants Help B Cell IgG Antibody Responses

KLH specific T_H clones were stimulated for 24 hr *in vitro* with syngeneic APC that had been pulsed with KLH, and the resulting supernatants were tested for helper activity by coculture with TNP-primed B cells and TNP-KLH. The supernatants derived from these helper clones supported predominantly IgG (<10% IgM) responses by syngeneic B cells to TNP-KLH (data not shown). Titrated numbers of intact T_H cells and titrated amounts of supernatant derived from these T_H cells were then compared in order to determine the relative efficiencies of help provided. The optimal response supported by intact T_H cells was approximately 5 µg/ml of anti-TNP antibody and occurred with 10^4 T cells / 1 ml culture; the background response in the absence of added T cells was 0.3 µg/ml. By comparison, the optimal response supported by clone 8-5 supernatant was 2 µg/ml at a 1/270 dilution of supernatant, which corresponds to the product of 2×10^3 T cells / 1 ml culture. Cloned T_H cells and their supernatants were thus approximately equivalent in their helper activity.

Antigen and MHC Specificity of T_H Factor

To test the specificity of T_H factor, supernatants prepared from clones of different antigen and MHC specificities were analyzed for antigen and MHC specificity in their function. Factor produced by clone 2-19-2 (specific for I-A^b+FGG) induced B10 cells to produce anti-TNP antibodies only in the presence of the specific antigen, TNP-FGG, and not in the presence of TNP-KLH. Reciprocally, supernatant from clone 8-5 (specific for I-A^b+KLH) induced B10 cells to produce anti-TNP antibody in response to TNP-KLH but not TNP-FGG (Table 1). These supernatants also showed the property of carrier-hapten linkage: supernatant from clone 8-5 (I-A^b+KLH) helped responses of B10 B cells to TNP-KLH but not to a mixture of KLH plus the hapten TNP on an irrelevant carrier (Table 1).

TABLE 1. Antigen specificity of B cell activation by T helper factor

Clone Supernatant	Clone Antigen Specificity	Antigen	Anti-TNP Antibody Response
2-19-2	FGG	TNP-FGG	+
		TNP-KLH	-
8-5	KLH	TNP-FGG	-
		TNP-KLH	+
		TNP-BSA + KLH	-

In order to determine if the helper factor (HF) released by T_H clones is MHC restricted as well as antigen specific in its function, supernatants were generated from clones which were specific for either KLH+I-A^b (clone 8-5) or KLH+I-A^k (clone A-12) and were tested for their ability to trigger B10 (I-A^b) or B10.A (I-A^k) B cells in response to TNP-KLH. Clone 8-5 HF was more effective in inducing IgG anti-TNP responses by B10 B cells than by MHC congenic B10.A B cells (Table 2). Similarly, A-12 HF stimulated B10.A but not B10 B cells (Table 2). B cell activation in this T cell-free system is therefore MHC-restricted. Supernatants generated by stimulating T_H clones with immobilized anti-CD3 in the absence of antigen or APC also showed both antigen specificity and MHC restriction.

TABLE 2. MHC restriction of B cell activation by T helper factor

| | | Anti-TNP Antibody Response | |
| | Clone | Source of B Cells | |
Clone Supernatant	MHC Restriction	B10 (I-A^b)	B10.A (I-A^k)
8-5	I-A^b	+	-
A-12	I-A^k	-	+

Requirement for Endogenous IL-4

Since the T_H clones employed in these studies have been shown to produce IL-4 (data not shown), the possible role of endogenous lymphokine in B cell responses supported by clone supernatants was examined. Affinity purified recombinant IL-4 (rIL-4) alone was not sufficient to trigger TNP-primed B10.BR cells to produce IgG anti-TNP in the presence of antigen (Table 3), whereas supernatant from clone A-8 supported an IgG anti-TNP response under the same conditions. A possible role of endogenous IL-4 was tested by adding titrated amounts of anti-IL-4 antibody into cultures containing B cells, clone supernatant and antigen. Anti-IL-4 antibody completely blocked responses (Table 3), whereas anti-IL-2 antibody did not inhibit the response of B10 B cells to 8-5 supernatant. IL-4 in clone supernatant is thus required for the activation of B cells by antigen specific helper T cell products.

TABLE 3. Role of IL-4 in B cell activation

Clone Supernatant	Added rIL-4	Anti-IL-4	Anti-IL-2	Anti-TNP B Cell Response
-	+	-	-	-
+	-	-	-	+
+	-	+	-	-
+	-	-	+	+

Affinity Purification of ASHF by Binding to Antibody Specific For a TCR Vβ Determinant

The antigen and MHC specificity of the help mediated by T_H clone supernatants closely mimicked the specificity of the intact T_H cells from which these supernatants were derived. Since the specificity of these T cells is apparently mediated by the αβ TCR heterodimer, experiments were designed to test whether the ASHF in Th cell supernatant was related to this αβ dimer. Supernatants were prepared from clones that expressed TCR Vβ8 (and therefore were reactive with the monoclonal antibody F23.1) or did not express Vβ8 (and therefore were F23.1 negative). These supernatants were then absorbed with Sepharose coupled with F23.1 or to control irrelevant antibody. This absorption removed substantial helper activity from the supernatants of F23.1$^+$ T_H clones, but had no effect on supernatants of F23.1⁻ clones (Table 4). The material which had been bound to F23.1-Sepharose was then recovered by acid elution and tested for helper activity in the presence of added rIL-2 plus rIL-4. Eluate from F23.1⁺ clone supernatants provided help for anti-TNP IgG responses, and this help was both antigen-specific and MHC-restricted (Table 5). The ASHF released by cloned T_H cells, in addition to functionally paralleling the specificity of the $\alpha\beta$ TCR, thus also expresses serologically defined TCR Vβ determinants.

TABLE 4. Absorption of ASHF with anti-TCR Vβ8 antibody

Clone Supernatant	F23.1 Expression By Th Clone	Absorbant	Anti-TNP B Cell Response
		None	+
10-5-17	+	F23-Sepharose	-
		BSA-Sepharose	+
		None	+
8-5	-	F23-Sepharose	+
		BSA-Sepharose	+

TABLE 5. Antigen and MHC specificity of helper factor eluted from anti-TCR antibody

Clone Supernatant	Eluate From	rIL-2+rIL-4	Antigen	Antibody Response Source of B Cells	
				B10	B10.A
None	-	+	TNP-KLH	-	-
10-5-17	BSA-Sepharose	+	TNP-KLH	-	-
	F23-Sepharose	-	TNP-KLH	-	-
		+	TNP-KLH	+	-
		+	TNP-FGG	-	-

DISCUSSION

The present study demonstrated that: 1) Antigen specific helper activity in the supernatants of T_H clones was capable of replacing intact T_H cells in the generation of TNP-specific IgG response. 2) The induction of B cell antibody responses by T_H cell supernatants was both antigen specific (carrier-hapten linked) and MHC-restricted, similar to some of the previously described ASHF (22-29). 3) B cell antibody responses require both an antigen-specific signal and a nonspecific lymphokine-mediated signal that synergize in their direct effect on B cells. 4) ASHF was affinity purified by binding to monoclonal antibody specific for a TCR VB8 determinant.

The specific signal provided to B cells by ASHF was both carrier-hapten linked and MHC restricted. This is consistent with a model in which hapten-specific B cells efficiently process and present the carrier determinants which are present on carrier-hapten conjugates (30, 31). The helper factor would then interact specifically with those B cells expressing the appropriate MHC product. Interaction of ASHF with cell surface Ia molecules on the B cell may lead to signal transduction through these Ia receptors. Lymphokine effects appear to synergize with antigen specific factors. IL-4 might function via its known ability to induce increased Ia density on B cells, thus facilitating the interaction with Ia-restricted T cell factor. Alternatively, antigen-specific factors may increase responsiveness to lymphokines. Populations of accessory cells in the responding B cell population may play a role in these interactions.

The antigen specificity and MHC restriction of ASHF in the present studies parallel precisely the specificity of intact cloned T_H cells, where this specificity is apparently mediated by the TCR $\alpha\beta$ heterodimer (32). Moreover, the antigen-specific helper activity contained in these supernatants was absorbed by immobilized antibody specific for TCR $V\beta8$ determinants (F23.1), and ASHF was recovered from this antibody which could support B cell responses in the presence of added recombinant lymphokines. In addition, it has recently been shown that the supernatants produced by T_H clones contain TCR $\alpha\beta$ dimers that can be metabolically labeled and immunoprecipitated by F23.1 (21). The ability to isolate a shed, secreted or proteolytically cleaved form of the TCR would offer a unique resource for the direct study of this receptor and its ligand specificity. In addition this system will provide an opportunity to study directly the interaction of specific and nonspecific helper signals in B cell activation.

SUMMARY

T helper (T_H) clones of different antigen specificities and MHC restriction were tested for their ability to produce soluble factors capable of providing help for B cell IgG antibody responses. T_H clone supernatants were generated by stimulation with specific antigen and antigen presenting cells (APC) or by stimulation with immobilized anti-CD3 antibody in the absence of antigen or APC. These supernatants contained helper activity that was antigen specific and MHC restricted, and paralleled the specificity of the intact T_H cells which is presumably mediated by the cell surface T cell receptor (TCR). In addition to the specific helper factor present in T_H clone supernatants, a role for nonspecific lymphokines was also identified. Although IL-4 alone was not sufficient to stimulate secretion of hapten specific IgG antibodies, anti-IL-4 antibody blocked the induction of antibody secretion by T_H cell supernatant. Thus, the stimulation of B cells to produce hapten specific IgG antibody requires at least two distinct signals: an antigen-specific T cell signal which is restricted by MHC products expressed on the B cells, and a nonspecific signal mediated at least in part by the lymphokine IL-4. The antigen-specific helper activity of T_H supernatants was specifically absorbed with antibody specific for TCR $V\beta$ determinants, and helper activity could be recovered by elution from this antibody. Affinity-purified helper factor was capable of acting together with recombinant lymphokines to support hapten-specific B cell antibody responses. Cell-free T_H cell products with both functional and serologic similarity to the cell surface TCR $\alpha\beta$ dimer are therefore able to provide a specific helper signal in the activation of B cell antibody responses.

REFERENCES

1. Singer, A., and Hodes, R. J. (1983): *Ann. Rev. Immunol.* 1:211-241.
2. Howard, M., and Paul, W. E. (1983): *Ann. Rev. Immunol.* 1:307-333.
3. Noelle, R. J., Snow, E. C., Uhr, J. W., and Vitetta, E. S. (1983): *Proc. Natl. Acad. Sci. USA* 80:6628-6631.
4. Kupfer, A., Swain, S. L., and Singer, S.J. (1987): *J. Exp. Med.* 165:1565-1580.
5. Sanders, V. M., Snyder, J.M., Uhr, J. W., and Vitetta, E. S. (1986): *J. Immunol.* 137:2395-2404.
6. DeFranco, A. L., Ashwell, J.D., Schwartz, R. H., and Paul, W. E. (1984): *J. Exp. Med.* 159:861-880.
7. Leclercq, L., Bismuth, G., and Theze, J. (1984): *Proc. Natl. Acad. Sci. USA* 81:6491-6495.
8. Hodes, R. J., and Singer, A. (1977): *Eur. J. Immunol.* 7:892-897.
9. Asano, Y., and Hodes, R. J. (1983): *J. Exp. Med.* 158:1178-1190.
10. Henkart, P., Henkart, M., Hodes, R. J., and Taplits, M. (1987): *Bioscience Reports* 7:345-353.
11. Taplits, M.S., Henkart, P.A., and Hodes, R.J. (1988): *J. Immunol.* 141:1-9.
12. Leo, O., Foo, M., Sachs, D. H., Samelson, L. E., and Bluestone, J. A. (1987): *Proc. Natl. Acad. Sci. USA* 84:1374-1378.
13. Ohara, J., and Paul, W. E. (1985): *Nature* 315:333-336.
14. Mosmann, T. H., Cherwinski, H., Bond, M. W., Geidlen, M., and Coffman, R. L. (1986): *J. Immunol.* 136:2348-2357.
15. Lake, P., Clark, E. A., Khorshidi, M., and Sunshine, G.H. (1979): *Eur. J. Immunol.* 9:875-886.
16. Staerz, U. D., Rammensee, H. -G., Benedetto, J. D., and Bevan, M. J. (1985): *J. Immunol.* 134:3994-4000.
17. Grabstein, K., Eiseman, J., Mochizuki, D., Shanebeck, K., Conlon, P., Hopp, T., March, C., and Gillis, S. (1986): *J. Exp. Med.* 163:1405-1414.
18. Guy, R., and Hodes, R. J. (1989): *J. Immunol.* 143:1433-1440.
19. Asano, Y., Singer, A., and Hodes, R. J. (1981): *J. Exp. Med.* 154:1100-1115.
20. Hathcock, K. S., Kenny, J. J., and Hodes, R. J. (1985): *Eur. J. Immunol.* 15:564-569.
21. Guy, R., Ullrich, S. J., Foo-Philips, M., Hathcock, K. S., Appella, E., and Hodes, R. J. (1989): *Science* 244:1477-1479.
22. Lifshitz, R., Apte, R. N., and Mozes, E. (1983): *Proc. Natl. Acad. Sci. USA* 80:5689-5693.
23. Krowka, J. F., Shiozawa, C., Diener, E., and Pilarski, L. M. (1986): *Transplantation* 42:162-167.
24. Dekruyff, R. H., Clayberger, C., and Cantor, H. (1983): *J. Exp. Med.* 158:1881-1894.
25. Azar, Y., Falk, P., Kagan, Y., and Ben-Sasson, S. Z. (1985): *J. Immunol.* 134:1717-1722.
26. Guy, R., and Ben-Sasson, S. Z. (1984): *Cell. Immunol.* 89:186-193.
27. Lonai, P., Puri, J., and Hammerling, G. (1981): *Proc. Natl. Acad. Sci. USA* 78:549-553.
28. Axelrode, O., and Mozes, E. (1987): *J. Immunogenetics* 14:109-115.
29. Shiozawa, C., Sewada, S., Inazawa, M., and Diener, E. (1984): *J. Immunol.* 132:1892-1899.
30. Rock, K. L., Benacerraf, B., and Abbas, A. K. (1984): *J. Exp. Med.* 160:1102-1113.
31. Malynn, B. A., Romeo, D. T., and Wortis, H. H. (1985): *J. Immunol.* 135:980-988.
32. Kronenberg, M., Siu, G., Hood, L. E., and Shastri, N. (1986): *Ann. Rev. Immunol.* 4:529-591.

Molecular Aspects of Immune Response and Infectious Diseases, edited by H. Kiyono, E. Jirillo, and C. DeSimone. Raven Press, Ltd., New York, © 1990.

15

Receptor Functions Associated with the Cell Surface I-J Molecule

T. Tada, Y. Asano, K. Sano, T. Komuro, T. Nakayama, and H. Kishimoto

Department of Immunology, Faculty of Medicine, University of Tokyo, 7-3-1 Hongo, Bunkyo-ku, Tokyo 113, Japan

INTRODUCTION

I-J is an enigmatic T cell surface molecule capable of changing its serological specificity according to the environmental MHC during the early ontogeny of T cells in the thymus (1-3). No I-J gene has been found in the I region of MHC where I-J was originally mapped (4), and thus, the early notion of I-J as a direct product of an MHC gene (5, 6) has been withheld. It is now suspected that I-J is a receptor like molecule adaptively expressed on T cells which recognizes MHC polymorphism.

Despite its ambiguous nature, the biological importance of I-J has been well documented. Early reports have demonstrated the association of I-J with antigen-specific suppressive T cell factors (TsF) and the requirement for I-J identity (I-J restriction) in suppressive cell interactions (6-8). More recently, it has been shown that monoclonal anti-I-J antibodies could inhibit the autologous and allogeneic mixed lymphocyte reaction (9), antigen-induced T cell proliferation and helper functions by acting on T cells but not on accessory cells (1, 10). The possibility that I-J is an idiotypic determinant of the T cell antigen receptor (TCR) has been excluded by experiments that the I-J does not comodulate with TCR/CD3 complex on the surface of cloned T cells treated with anti-CD3 antibody (10). In addition, we have found that the treatment of T cells with anti-I-J can inhibit the early increase of intracellular Ca^{2+} ions induced by the stimulation with antigen and antigen-presenting cells (APC) (Asano *et al.*, manuscript in preparation). The mode of inhibition of Ca^{2+} influx is very similar to that caused by the interaction with T suppressor (Ts) cells, which is the initial event in the suppressive cell interaction (11). The molecular nature of I-J polypeptide has also been investigated to certain extent to show some unique biochemical properties (12). The present report is to describe some functional and molecular properties of the I-J polypeptide in conjunction with the suppression phenomena induced through the cell surface I-J molecule.

EPIGENETIC EXPRESSION OF I-J EPITOPE ON T CELL CLONES DERIVED FROM DIFFERENT ORIGINS

We have established a large number of IL-2-dependent T cell clones from C3H (H-2^k), B6 (H-2^b), B10, (C3H x B6)F_1, $F_1 \rightarrow$ C3H, $F_1 \rightarrow$ B6, and B6 $\rightarrow$ F_1 radiation bone marrow chimeras (10). They are maintained with periodical stimulation with antigen [keyhole limpet hemocyanin (KLH) or fowl gamma globulin (FGG)] and APC of H-2^k or H-2^b followed by propagation in IL-2 containing medium. Most of them are CD4+ T_H or Ts, while two clones are CD8+ Ts. The CD4+ Ts clone is defined by the criteria where the clone does not produce both IL-2 and IL-4, has no detectable helper activity in the *in vitro* antibody response, and exerts a strong inhibitory activity on the antibody response of MHC-compatible T_H and B cells. Table 1 is the list of these T cell clones used in the subsequent studies.

Several of these T cell clones have been found to express I-J^k epitope detected by an anti-I-J^k antibody JK-10. This antibody is the product of a hybridoma derived from spleen cells of B10.A(3R) immunized with B10.A(5R) differing only in the I-J phenotype, and has been shown to absorb TsF from H-2^k but not from H-2^b mice. The presence of I-J^k on T cell clones was determined by the inhibition of antigen-induced proliferation and helper function by the antibody or by the immunofluorescent cell surface staining with fluorescinated JK-10.

The I-J^k expression on these T cell clones is generally associated with their MHC-restriction specificity (Table 1). A^k- and E^k-restricted clones are I-J^k positive regardless of their haplotype origin. Notable examples are clones from B6 $\rightarrow$ F_1 chimeras having either A^k or E^k restriction specificity. They express I-J^k which are not normally expressed on B6-derived T cell clones. The expression is regardless of their functions; both H-2^k-restricted T_H and Ts clones have the identical I-J^k epitope. One CD8+ Ts clone from C3H with an ability to product TsF is also positive.

However, the I-J^k expression does not always correlate with the MHC restriction specificity. Two T cell clones of 5R origin, one having A^b-restriction and the other having E^k-restriction specificities, are I-J^k positive, whereas an A^b-restricted T cell clone derived from 3R is negative by all means. These results confirm our previous findings that I-J^k is epigenetically expressed on chimeric T cells according to the host environment (1, 2), and that 3R and 5R differ in the I-J phenotype regardless of the similarity of their I region DNA sequence.

I-J AS A RECEPTOR-LIKE MOLECULE TRANSDUCING A NEGATIVE SIGNAL

It has been reported that monoclonal anti-I-J antibodies are capable of inhibiting helper activity and antigen-induced proliferative response of normal T cells and T cell clones (1, 10). To delineate the mechanism of anti-I-J-induced suppression,

TABLE 1. Expression of I-J^k epitope on T cell clones

Code	Origin	Specificity	Function		I-J^k Expression
MS-2	C3H	A^k	Th		+
9-5	F$_1$^{b}	A^k + KLH		Ts	+
9-16	F$_1$	E^k + KLH	Th		+
28-4	F$_1$	A^k + KLH	Th		+
23-1-8	F$_1$ → C3H	A^k + KLH	Th		+
23-2	F$_1$ → C3H	E^k + KLH	Th		+
25-11-20	B$_6$ → F$_1$	A^k + KLH		Ts	+
25-18-5	B$_6$ → F$_1$	E^k + KLH		Ts	+
2-19-2	B10	A^b + FGG, A^{bm12}	Th		-
8-4	F$_1$	A^b + KLH		Ts	-
8-5	F$_1$	A^b + KLH	Th		-
24-2	F$_1$ → B6	A^b + KLH	Th		-
24-15-1	F$_1$ → B6	A^b	Th		-
40-5	B10.A(5R)	E^k + KLH		Ts	+
40-12	B10.A(5R)	A^b + KLH		Ts	+
44-11	B10.A(3R)	A^b + KLH		Ts	-
3D10[a]	C3H	A^k + KLH		Ts	+
13G2[a]	B6	A^b + Casein		Ts	-

[a]L3T4$^-$, Ly-2$^+$
[b]B6C3F$_1$

we have studied the effect of anti-I-J on the intracellular signal transduction of T cells induced by antigenic stimulation.

T cell clones were labeled with Ca^{2+}-sensitive fluorophore Fura 2AM. The cells were stimulated with antigen and APC or other mitogenic stimuli which induce the increase in the intracellular Ca^{2+} ([Ca^{2+}]i), which was measurable by an stopped-flow fluorometry (11). The anti-I-J antibodies were applied to the cells before the mitogenic stimulation.

As shown in Figure 1, the treatment of a T$_H$ clone 23-1-8, which had been derived from F$_1$ → C3H chimera and is restricted to A^k molecule, with anti-I-J^k (JK-10) resulted in the inhibition of Ca^{2+} influx which was induced by antigen and APC. The inhibition was comparable to that induced by anti-CD4 (anti-L3T4). Anti-I-J^b (WF8.D2.4, kindly provided by Dr. C. Waltenbough) had no effect on this A^k-restricted T$_H$ clone. However, if the same treatments were applied to an A^b-restricted Th clone 8-5 derived from H-2^{kxb}F$_1$, anti-I-J^b could inhibit the Ca^{2+}

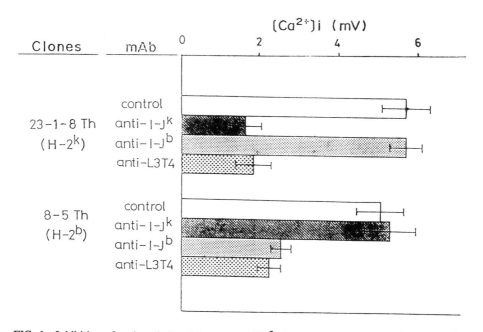

FIG. 1. Inhibition of antigen-induced increase of $[Ca^{2+}]i$ by the treatment of $H-2^k$- and $H-2^b$-restricted T cell clones with anti-I-J antibodies. The Th clone 23-1-8 is derived from KLH-primed $(C3H \times B6)F_1$ C3H chimera and restricted to $H-2^k$. The treatment with anti-I-J^k (JK-10) but not with anti-I-J^b (WF8.D2.4) inhibited the Ca^{2+} response against the subsequent stimulation with KLH and APC. If another Th clone 8-5, derived from $(C3H \times B6)F_1$ was treated by the same antibodies, anti-I-J^b but not anti-I-J^k could selectively inhibit the Ca^{2+} response. Since the genotype of these clones is the same, the result indicates that functional I-J phenotypes of these clones are mutually excluded. Some other properties of the anti-I-J-induced suppression of Ca^{2+} responses and discussed in the text.

response of this clone to a degree comparable to that induced by anti-CD4. Anti-I-J^k was ineffective for this A^b-restricted clone. Since both these clones have the same F_1 genotype, it is clear that I-J phenotype is not primarily determined by the H-2 genotype of the cells, and that the expression of I-J^k and I-J^b is mutually excluded in F_1 T cell clones.

It was further found that intact anti-I-J, but not the monovalent Fab fragment of anti-I-J was able to inhibit the antigen-induced Ca^{2+} influx. The addition of anti-mouse Ig antibodies to the cells treated with the fragment resulted in the inhibition of Ca^{2+} influx. Thus, the inhibitory effect of anti-I-J is not merely a blocking of a site involved in the antigen-recognition but due to the induction of an active intracellular process by the ligation of surface I-J molecules.

Furthermore, the inhibitory effect of anti-I-J was directed only to the activation signal induced through the TCR $\alpha\beta$ heterodimer. The increase of $[Ca^{2+}]i$ induced by Con A or by anti-CD3 was not inhibitable by anti-I-J. The Ca^{2+} influx induced by a monoclonal anti-TCR $\alpha\beta$ heterodimer (H57-597, kindly provided by Dr. R.T. Kubo) was, however, inhibitable by the same anti-I-J. These results led us to suspect that I-J is involved in a very early membrane process subsequent to the recognition of antigen via the TCR heterodimer, while the subsequent intracellular signal transduction induced through the CD3 complex is not inhibitable. It is not known whether there is an intermedialy messenger between TCR heterodimer and CD3, but the I-J derived inhibitory signal seems to interfere with the process present in between TCR heterodimer and CD3. Alternatively, the signals transduced by specific ligand and anti-CD3 may utilize different activation pathways for Ca^{2+} influx.

MOLECULAR CHARACTERIZATION OF I-J

We have recently identified the I-J molecule as a dimeric glycoprotein of M.W. 84 - 88 kD composed of 43 - 44 kD subunit in two dimensional (2D, reducing/nonreducing) gel analysis (12). T cell clones were surface labeled with ^{125}I, lysed in 1% NP-40, and precipitated with anti-I-J^k (JK-10) or control antibodies. The materials were analyzed by one or 2D SDS-polyacrylamide gel and nonequilibrated pH gradient electrophoresis (NEPHGE).

Figure 2 illustrates the electrophoretic identification of I-J molecule in the lysate of a T cell clone MS-S2 in 2D gel as a distinct molecule from TCR $\alpha\beta$ heterodimer. The anti-I-J precipitated a 44 kD molecule migrating as an off-diagonal spot. A monoclonal IgG_{2a} of anti-$V_{\beta 8}$, which does not react with TCR of this T cell clone, precipitated no comparable molecules. I-J is clearly distinguishable from TCR α and β chains (Figure 2c) which were precipitated with a rabbit polyvalent anti-TCR antiserum (6623, kindly provided by Dr. R. T. Kubo). The off-diagonal 44 kD molecule is apparently derived from a 86 kD dimer. Figure 2d shows the result of sequential immunoprecipitation with anti-TCR and anti-I-J, where the 44 kD molecule is still detectable after preclearance with anti-TCR.

We have studied the expression of immunoprecipitable I-J^k molecules on various T cell clones, normal and malignant cells. It was confirmed that most of A^k- and E^k-restricted T cell clones derived from F_1 and chimeric animals showed the positive I-J^k immunoprecipitation, whereas A^b-restricted clones of the similar origins were negative. A 5R clone but not 3R clone having A^b-restriction showed a positive immunoprecipitation. Thus, the I-J molecule identifiable by gel electrophoresis has the same specificity as that detected by functional assays.

In the NEPHGE analysis, the I-J subunit migrates to a relatively acidic position of pH 5.0 to 6.0 which is distinguishable from TCR α and β chains, and from class I heavy chains. The relatively homogeneous isoelectric point of I-J molecule in NEPHGE suggests that the I-J on the cell surface may be a homodimer, but this has not been formally proven. Although in some T cell clones, on-diagonal spot of monomeric 44 kD was detected, only the dimeric form was generally detectable in most T cell clones. The I-J was found to be a lightly glycosilated polypeptide, as the treatment with endo-β-N-acetyl glucosaminidase F (endo F) reduced the M.W. of the subunit to 41 KDa which was larger than those of TCR α and β chains after the identical endo F treatment. The M.W. microheterogeneity observed among T cell clones may be due to the difference in glycosilation.

The molecular identity of I-J has been studied in comparison with various other T cell membrane molecules. It has been shown that I-J is different from 90 kD disulfide-linked dimeric molecule such as A1 and YE1/48 antigen of EL4 (13, 14), and putative mouse CD28 (15). Apparently, it is different from usual class I antigen, which sometimes form dimers in the extraction process, because of its extremely small quantity on the cell surface and of its mutually excluded expression

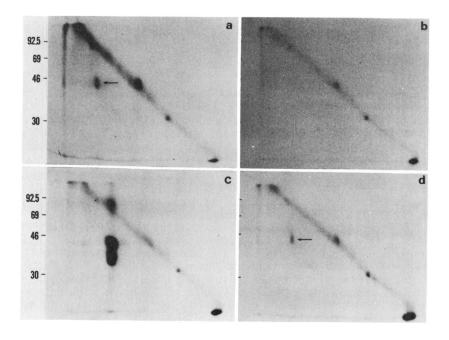

FIG. 2. Two-dimensional SDS-polyacrylamide gel electrophoresis (SDS-PAGE) of I-J molecule and TCR from a T cell clone MS-S2. This clone is an IL-2-dependent I-A^k-autoreactive T cell clone established from C3H (H-2^k). ^{125}I-surface labeled cells were solubilized in isotonic buffer containing 1% NP-40. Immunoprecipitates were prepared with (a) JK10-23 (anti-I-J^k mAb, IgG$_{2a}$), (b) F23.1 (an irrelevant anti-TCR V$_{\beta 8}$), (c) 6623 (pan-reactive rabbit anti-TCR antiserum), and (d) JK10-23 after preclearance with 6623. Precipitates were analyzed by two-dimensional (nonreducing/reducing) SDS-PAGE. Note an off-diagonal spot (an arrow in a and d) of 44kD which is derived from a Mr 86 kD molecule, and is distinct from TCR α and β chains (c).

in F$_1$ T cells (1). The adaptive expression in chimeric animals also suggest that I-J is different from conventional class I.

We have recently produced xenogeneic (rat) monoclonal antibodies against the I-J molecule precipitated by JK-10, and studied the molecules precipitable by these antibodies by gel electrophoresis. These rat antibodies stained thymocytes and spleen cells of various H-2 congeneic and recombinant strains, the pattern of which do not fit previously known mouse MHC polymorphism. In addition, they precipitated multiple molecules from T cell clones and normal thymocytes. Thus, the antibodies are detecting epitopes shared by a set of proteins. At least, one of these molecules was a class I, suggesting that I-J may carry an epitope cross-reactive with a class I molecule. Several other spots are distinct from class I molecules with respect to M.W. and the isoelectric point. We are currently studying to identify the molecule corresponding to I-J in such gels, and to clone the gene encoding the I-J and related molecules.

DISCUSSION

The above findings indicate that I-J is a novel dimeric molecule expressed on antigen-specific T cells and T cell clones. Because of its adaptive generation on T cells in radiation bone marrow chimeras and of its association with the acquired restriction specificity, it is likely to be a receptor-like molecule. It is different from conventional TCR α and β chains, but produces a negative signal to prevent the Ca^{2+} influx caused by the recognition of antigen through TCR heterodimer. The pattern of inhibition of Ca^{2+} influx in T_H cells is very similar to that induced by the interaction with activated Ts cells. In view of the long history of I-J in conjunction with the suppressor phenomena, we think that I-J is a receptor on various cell types in the suppressor pathway that mediates suppressive cell interactions. The anti-I-J antibody acts as an agonist for the suppressor signal given to the target cells.

The molecular nature of the I-J is still unknown. The electrophoretic behavious resembles with that of class I, however, it is different from known conventional class I antigens. The quantity as well as the selective expression only in restricted T cell clones in F_1 also distinguishes it from known class I. Isoelectric point of I-J is different from that of general class I molecules. Whether it is a modified class I or a new molecule of a family of related proteins should be investigated. Further molecular studies will reveal the true figure of these enigmatic but biologically important molecule.

ACKNOWLEDGEMENTS

The work presented in this paper has been supported by the grants from the Ministry of Education, Culture and Science, and Agency of Science and Technology, Japan. The authors are grateful for the secretarial help by Ms. Yoko Yamaguchi.

REFERENCES

1. Asano, Y., Nakayama, T., Kubo, M., Yagi, J., and Tada, T. (1987): *J. Exp. Med.* 166:1613-1623.
2. Uracz, W., Asano, Y., Abe, R., and Tada, T. (1986): *Nature* 316:741-743.
3. Sumida, T., Sado, T., Kojima, M., Ono, H., Kamisaku, K., and Taniguchi, M. (1985): *Nature* 316:738-741.
4. Steinmetz, M., Minard, K., Horvath, S., McNicholas, J., Frelinger, J., Wake, C., Long, E., Mach, B., and Hood, L. (1976): *Nature* 300:35-42.
5. Murphy, D. B., Herzenberg, L. A., Okumura, K., Herzenberg, L. A., and McDevitt, H. (1976): *J. Exp. Med.* 144:699-712.
6. Tada, T., Taniguchi, M., and David, C. S. (1976): *J. Exp. Med.* 144:713-723.
7. Dorf, M. E., and Benacerraf, B. (1985): *Immunol. Rev.* 83:23-40.
8. Tada, T., and Okumura, K. (1979): *Adv. Immunol.* 28:1-87.
9. Uracz, W., Abe, R., and Tada, T. (1985): *Proc. Natl. Acad. Sci. USA* 82:2905-2909.
10. Nakayama, T., Kubo, R. T., Kubo, M., Fujisawa, I., Kishimoto, H., Asano, Y., and Tada, T. (1988): *Eur. J. Immunol.* 18:761-765.
11. Utsunomiya, N., Nakanishi, M., Arata, Y., Kubo, M., Asano, Y., and Tada, T. (1989): *Int. Immunol.* 1:460-463.

12. Nakayama, T., Kubo, R. T., Kishimoto, H., Asano, Y., and Tada, T. (1989): *Int. Immunol.* 1:50-58.
13. Nagasaw, R., Cross, J., Kanagawa, O., Townsend, K., Laner, L. L., Chiller, J., and Allison, J. A. (1987): *J. Immunol.* 138:815-824.
14. Chan, P. -Y., and Takei, F. (1988): *J. Immunol.* 140:161-169.
15. Yokoyama, W. M., Koning, F., Kehn, P. J., Pereira, G. M. B., Stingl, G., Goligan, J. E., and Shevach, E. M. (1988): *J. Immunol.* 141:369-376.

Molecular Aspects of Immune Response and Infectious Diseases, edited by H. Kiyono, E. Jirillo, and C. DeSimone. Raven Press, Ltd., New York, © 1990.

16

Differentiation of an Interleukin 3-Dependent Precursor Cell into Myeloid Cells as Well as B Lymphocytes

T. Kinashi*, K. Tashiro*, K. H. Lee*, K. Inaba+, K. Toyama*, R. Palacios§, and T. Honjo*

The Department of Medical Chemistry, Faculty of Medicine, +Department of Zoology, Faculty of Science, Kyoto University, Kyoto 606, Japan, and §Basel Institute for Immunology, Basel, Switzerland

INTRODUCTION

T and B lymphocytes are believed to differentiate from a common precursor cell that itself is derived from a bone marrow stem cell. One of the most interesting features of lymphocyte differentiation is its association with DNA rearrangement in the immunoglobulin loci of B lymphocytes or in the T cell receptor loci of T lymphocytes. The V-D-J recombination that brings the variable (V), diversity (D) and joining (J) segments together to form a complete V gene is a decisive step of the B or T cell differentiation and, thus, serves as a genetic marker of commitment to either B or T lineage (1,2).

To investigate regulation of the decisive step of B-cell differentiation, it is important to establish an *in vitro* system that allows induction of the V-D-J and V-J recombination in a cell line containing the germ-line context of the immunoglobulin gene. Establishment of interleukin (IL)-3-dependent progenitor cell lines, each of which can differentiate *in vivo* into either B or T lymphocytes (3,4) provided unique model systems for molecular biological studies on cellular commitment.

We report here the IL-3-dependent LyD9 progenitor clone has differentiated into mature B cells and myeloid cells *in vitro* when cocultured with bone marrow stroma cells. We will also describe establishment of an IL-4-dependent clone (K-4) that was derived from induced LyD9 cells. The K-4 clone is a multipotential intermediate in differentiation from the LyD9 clone to B cells and myeloid cells.

MATERIALS AND METHODS

Animals and Cells

IL-3-dependent cell lines (LyD9) were established from a 4-week-old CBA/J mouse (5). ST-2 stromal cell line (6) established from Whitlock-Witte type bone marrow culture was provided by Dr. S. Nishikawa (Kumamoto Univ.).

Induction with Bone Marrow Stroma Cells

Bone marrow stroma cells were prepared as described (7). LyD9 cells (1 x 10^5) were mixed and cocultured with bone marrow stroma cells (5 x 10^5) as described (8). After 10 days of culture, cells were harvested for immunofluorescence staining with polyclonal rabbit anti-murine IgM or IgG antibody or with MB86 monoclonal anti-μ chain antibody (9).

Establishment of K-4, K-GM and LS-1 Cells

Induced LyD9 cells (5 x 10^5) which had been cocultured with bone marrow stroma cells were collected and recultured in the complete medium containing 1 mg/ml G418 (Sigma) supplemented with 10 U/ml rIL-4 or 20 U/ml rGM-CSF. rIL-4 or rGM-CSF was added to the culture medium every third day. The outgrowth of cells became apparent in two weeks. The LS-1 clone was established as follows: Induced LyD9 cells (5 x 10^5/ml) were transferred and maintained on a monolayer of ST-2 cells in the complete medium supplemented with 25 μg/ml LPS and 1 mg/ml G418. After 4 weeks the growing cells were subcloned with the limiting dilution procedure using round-bottom microtiter plates precoated with ST-2 cells. One of the outgrown cells (LS-1) were expanded and maintained on a monolayer of ST-2 in the complete medium supplemented with 25 μg/ml LPS.

Morphological Analysis

Cytocentrifuge preparations of cells were stained with May-Grünwald-Giemsa. Nonspecific esterase granules were detected with α-naphthyl butyrate or chloroacetate method. Peroxidase granules were detected as described (10).

RESULTS

Differentiation of LyD9 Cells by Coculture with Bone Marrow Stroma Cells

We cocultured LyD9 cells with bone marrow stroma cells. LyD9 cells were loosely associated with the stroma cells and grew on their surface. After 10 days of the culture, LyD9 cells formed a monolayer sheet over the stroma cell layer, and floating cells increased in number. Few floating cells appears without the addition of LyD9 cells. The cocultured LyD9 cells were analyzed with flow cytometry after staining with antibodies against IgM, B220, and Thy-1.2. The expression of the B-220 antigen increased during coculture (Figure 1A), but no Thy-1.2-positive

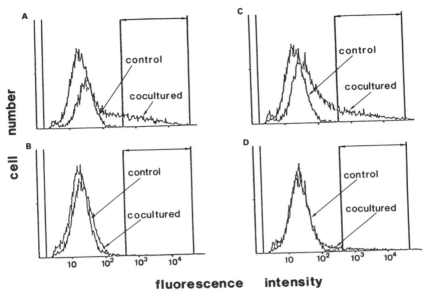

fluorescence   intensity

FIG. 1. Induction of the surface IgM on LyD9 cells by the coculture with bone marrow accessory cells. LyD9 cells were cocultured with bone marrow accessory cells. After 10 days of culture, cells were harvested for immunofluorescence staining with anti-B220 antibody (A), anti-Thy-1.2 antibody (B), polyclonal anti-murine IgM antibody (C), or MB86 monoclonal anti-μ chain antibody (D). The anti-μ chain antibody was used in C does not distinguish *j* and *n* allotypes, whereas the one used in (D) recognizes the *n* allotype but not *j* allotype. Uninduced LyD9 cells were used as a negative control. Stained cells were analyzed by a fluorescence-activated cell sorter (ABCAS100).

cells appeared (Figure 1B). The uninduced LyD9 cells were negative for surface IgM, but 17% of the induced LyD9 cells were stained with anti-IgM (Figure 1C). We used the bone marrow stroma cells of NZB mice, which have the IgM molecule of *n* allotype, so that we could distinguish IgM-bearing cells of LyD9 (*j* allotype) from those of NZB mice (*n* allotype) with use of the MB86 monoclonal antibody (9). IgM-bearing cells derived from NZB mice were few (at most 4%) (Figure 1D), indicating that LyD9 cells differentiated *in vitro* with high frequency. The number of cells producing IgM increased greatly when LyD9 cells were treated beforehand with 5-azacytidine (11).

Then we stained the induced LyD9 with anti-IgG antibody to see whether or not these cells also underwent class switch to produce IgG antibody. About 10% of LyD9 cells were IgG-positive, whereas essentially no IgG-bearing cells were found in the control culture with LyD9 cells. The production of IgM and IgG was further confirmed by measuring the amounts of IgM and IgG in the supernatant of the coculture (Table 1). After a 10 day coculture with stroma cells, 3.2 μg of IgM and 1.4 μg of IgG per ml were secreted by LyD9 cells. Negligible amounts of immunoglobulin were found in supernatants of stroma cells without LyD9.

To confirm the expression of immunoglobulin by induced LyD9 cells, we measured immunoglobulin mRNA in LyD9 cells cocultured with bone marrow stroma cells. RNA blot hybridization showed that the C_μ and C_κ transcripts in differentiated LyD9 were full-length mRNAs and not sterile transcripts of the immunoglobulin C genes (11).

TABLE 1. Production of IgM and IgG by LyD9 cells cocultured with bone marrow stroma cells

Presence of LyD9	Isotype and Level of Immunoglobulin (ng/ml)	
	IgM	IgG
+	3,200	1,400
-	<1	<8

Culture supernatants of day 10 coculture described in Materials and Methods were assayed for Ig by ELISA.

Random V-D-J Recombination

We also tested whether these IgM-bearing cells had rearranged selected V_H and V_K segments of the immunoglobulin gene. Southern blot filters of digested DNA from induced LyD9 cells that were 15% IgM positive were hybridized with J_H or J_K probe together with the C_K probe as an internal reference (Figure 2A, lanes 1-4). We did not find any discrete rearranged bands hybridized with either the J_H or J_K probe. After longer exposure (Figure 2B, lanes 1-4) smears of both larger and smaller sizes appeared, and the germ-line J_H or J_K bands relative to that of the C_K band decreased to 61% and 65%, respectively, at day 9 of coculture as compared with that in uninduced LyD9 cells.

These results indicate that the J_H and J_K segments were associated with heterogenous V_H and V_K segments to yield J_H and J_K fragments of different lengths. The results excluded the possibility that the coculture procedure selected preexisting IgM-bearing clones in LyD9 cells. No rearrangement at T-cell receptor loci occurred in induced LyD9 as the relative intensity of the germ-line J_α and J_β segments was unchanged (Figure 2A, lanes 5-8), and no significant smears appeared even after a long exposure (Figure 2B, lanes 5-8). No rearrangement of the J_γ segment was found in induced LyD9 cells (data not shown).

Differentiation of the LyD9 Clone into Myeloid Cells as well as B Lymphocytes

Morphological and cytochemical studies on induced LyD9 cells showed that induced LyD9 cells contained not only lymphoid cells but also myeloid cells (Figure 3a and b). Some of induced LyD9 cells contained nonspecific esterase activity. Peroxidase-staining was weak but significant (data not shown). The frequency of myeloid cells was roughly proportional to the frequency of Mac-1+ cells (26%) determined by the FACS analysis (12). The culture of stroma cells without the LyD9 cells, however, did not give rise to either lymphoid or myeloid cells.

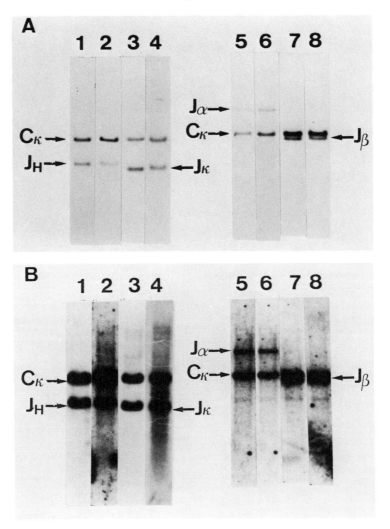

FIG. 2. Southern blot analysis of immunoglobulin gene loci and T-cell receptor loci in DNA of induced LyD9 cells. DNA was extracted from LyD9 cells cocultured with bone marrow stroma cells for 9 days, 15% of which expressed IgM on their surface, and was digested with *Xba*I. Since the *Xba*I site is between the J_K and C_K genes, the size of the C_K fragments should not be changed by the immunoglobulin gene recombination. Uninduced LyD9 DNAs were used as controls. Filters were exposed briefly to quantitate relative intensity of bands (A) and longer to see whether smeary bands appeared (B). Origins of DNA used are (i) uninduced LyD9 in lanes 1, 3, 5, and 7 and (ii) induced LyD9 in lanes 2, 4, 6, and 8. Probes used are (i) J_H and C_K (internal control) probes in lanes 1 and 2, (ii) J_K and C_K probes in lanes 3 and 4, (iii) J_α and C_K probes in lanes 5 and 6, and (iv) J_β and C_K probes in lanes 7 and 8. The germ-line *Xba*I fragments of the C_K (5.8 kb), J_H (3.8 kb), J_K (3.4 kb), J_α (9.0 kb), and J_β (5.3 kb) probes are indicated by arrows. Taken from Kinashi *et al.* (1989).

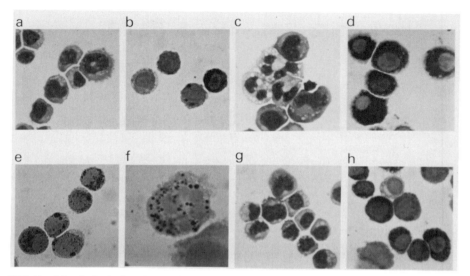

FIG. 3. Morphological and cytochemical analyses of the LyD9 clone and its derivatives. Cytocentrifuge preparations of induced LyD9 (a,b), LS-1 (c-f) and induced K-4 (g,h) were stained with May-Grünwald-Giemsa (a,c,g), for α-naphthyl-butyrate esterase (b,d,h), for chloroacetate esterase (e) and for peroxidase (f) as described (10). The magnification is X1,000 in (f) and X400 in the others. LS-1, LyD9 and K-4 cells were grown in media containing GM-CSF, IL-3 and IL-4, respectively.

TABLE 2. Response of LyD9 and its derivatives to growth factors

Growth Factors	Cell line tested and ^{3}H-thymidine (cpm) incorporation			
	LyD9	K-4	LS-1	K-GM
IL-1	60	180	0	580
IL-2	300	270	0	180
IL-3	26,200	30,000	35,500	19,800
IL-4	1,090	31,200	17,500	3,860
IL-5	0	730	5,410	60
IL-6	0	840	200	270
GM-CSF	0	1,110	45,100	36,500
M-CSF	0	660	26,400	0
G-CSF	0	550	30,800	460

Cells (4 x 10^4) were incubated in microplate wells with the complete medium (200 μl) containing growth factors indicated. The concentration of each growth factor was chosen so that the maximal plateau level of proliferative response is obtained. ^{3}H-Thymidine (0.5 μCi) was added to each culture well during the last 6 hours of the 48-hour incubation. Radioactivities incorporated into cells were measured by filtration and acid wash. The data are the mean of triplicate plates. The standard error was less than 10% of the mean throughout samples. Purified recombinant (r) human IL-1α and IL-2 were provided by Dainippon Pharmaceutical Company and Takeda Pharmaceutical Company (Japan), respectively. Purified murine rIL-3 was provided by DNAX Research Institute. Mouse rIL-4 and rIL-5 were obtained from X63 Ag8 myeloma cells transfected with IL-4 and IL-5 cDNAs. Purified human rIL-6 and murine recombinant GM-CSF were provided by Dr. T. Hirano (Osaka Univ.) and Dr. T. Sudo (Toray Basic Research Institute), respectively. Purified rG-CSF and human rM-CSF were provided by Dr. S. Nagata (Osaka Bioscience Institute).

Establishment of GM-CSF-Dependent Clones From Induced LyD9 Cells

Induced LyD9 cells harvested after 10 days of the coculture with stroma cells were transferred onto a stromal cell line ST-2, known to support both B lymphopoiesis and myelopoiesis from bone marrow progenitor cells (6). Stroma cell (ST-2)-dependent clones were established from this culture. Uninduced LyD9 cells could not survive on the ST-2 cell and died within a week. One of such clones, LS-1 was studied extensively.

GM-CSF-dependent clones were also established from induced LyD9 cells by repeated cloning in GM-CSF. One of these clones called K-GM had surface phenotypes similar to those of the LS-1 clone (Mac-1+, B220- and IgM-). The surface profiles of LS-1 and K-GM are consistent with those of myeloid lineage cells. Southern blot hybridization confirmed that both LS-1 and K-GM contained the same integration profile of the Neo^r gene as the parental LyD9 clone.

LS-1 proliferated well in the presence of either IL-3, IL-4, GM-CSF, M-CSF or G-CSF without ST-2 cells. However, neither IL-1, IL-2, IL-5 nor IL-6 could support the growth of LS-1 (Table 2). In fact, the LS-1 cells were also maintained in GM-CSF. K-GM grew not only in GM-CSF but also in IL-3, and to a lesser extent in IL-4.

Morphological Evidence That LS-1 and K-GM are Myeloid Lineage Cells

The LS-1 cells cultured in the presence of G-CSF and M-CSF contained cells similar to neutrophils and macrophages, respectively. Both macrophage- and neutrophil-like cells appeared in the LS-1 cells cultured in the presence of GM-CSF (Figure 3 c-f). The LS-1 cells expressed high levels of nonspecific esterases. Peroxidase-containing granules were found in neutrophil-like cells of the LS-1 cells, and also in macrophage-like cells albeit in lesser amounts. The K-GM cells contained both macrophage- and granulocyte-like cells which expressed non-specific esterases and peroxidase (data not shown). Typical macrophages and granulocytes appeared more frequently in the LS-1 cells and the K-GM cells grown in soft-agar cultures than in suspension cultures. Furthermore, PMA-treated LS-1 cells showed a strong non-specific phagocytosis activity. These results indicate that the LS-1 and K-GM clones belong to the granulocyte/macrophage lineage.

Involvement of IL-4 and LFA-1

Although neither IL-4 nor IL-5 supported differentiation of LyD9 cells into B cells, the addition of an anti-IL-4 antibody blocked proliferation and differentiation of LyD9 cells in coculture with stroma cells (Table 3). It is likely that proliferation and differentiation of LyD9 cells require some unknown growth factor or factors in addition to IL-4. An anti-IL-5 antibody did not affect differentiation of LyD9 cells (data not shown). The addition of an anti-LFA-1 antibody strongly inhibited proliferation and differentiation of LyD9 cells. LFA-1 belongs to the integrin family and contributes to cell-cell adhesion by interaction with intercellular adhesion molecule-1 (ICAM-1). LyD9 and stroma cells may require direct contact with each other. LyD9 cells actually grow with direct contact with stroma cells when we look at the cells under a microscope. It is worth noting that this amount

TABLE 3. Effects of antibodies on differentiation of LyD9 cells by coculture with bone marrow stroma cells

Antibodies Added	Numbers of cells (X10^{-3}/well)	IgM$^+$ cells (%)
Anti-IL-4	3.3	0
Anti-LFA-1	5.4	<2.5
Anti-B220	28.3	9.0
Anti-Mac-1	19.3	6.1
None	23.7	8.2

These antibodies in hybridoma culture supernatant were added to the coculture in a 1:9 (vol/vol) ratio (10% final volume) for 7 days, which did not affect proliferation of LyD9 in the presence of IL-3.

of antibodies did not affect proliferation of LyD9 cells in the presence of IL-3. Antibodies against other surface markers like B220 or Mac-1 did not affect differentiation and proliferation significantly. When these results are considered together, one concludes that LyD9 cells may be able to receive growth factors only when they have direct contact with stroma cells because the factor is in low concentration or because direct contact of cells stimulates production of these factors or their receptors.

Establishment of IL-4-Dependent Clones From Induced LyD9 Cells

We, therefore, attempted to isolate a possible intermediate cell between LyD9 and B cells by culturing induced LyD9 cells with IL-4. Several IL-4-dependent clones were established by repeated cloning of induced LyD9 cells in the presence of IL-4. Surface phenotypes of one of these clones, K-4 were almost identical to those of LyD9 (5) except that expression of the B220 antigen was about 2-fold augmented. The K-4 clone was certainly derived from the LyD9 clone because K-4 had the same integration pattern of the Neo^r gene as the parental LyD9 clone used.

We compared the growth response profile of the parental LyD9 and K-4 clones to various recombinant soluble factors [IL-1, IL-2, IL-3, IL-4, IL-5, IL-6, GM-CSF, M-CSF and G-CSF] (Table 2). LyD9 cells grew in IL-3, and responded to IL-4, albeit slightly and temporarily. On the other hand, K-4 cells were maintained in the medium containing either IL-4 or IL-3, and responded to IL-4 as strongly as IL-3. K-4 did not proliferate in IL-5, IL-6 or GM-CSF although weak responses to these factors were observed.

Differentiation of the K-4 Clone into Myeloid as well as B Lymphocytes

We examined whether the differentiation capacity into myeloid cells as well as B cells is maintained by the K-4 clone. K-4 cells were subjected to surface staining after coculture with bone marrow stroma cells under conditions known to promote B cell differentiation. The proportions of induced K-4 cells which strongly expressed the IgM, B220, and Mac-1 antigens were similar (13%, 22%, 26%, respectively) to those for the induced LyD9 clone. Morphological studies identified

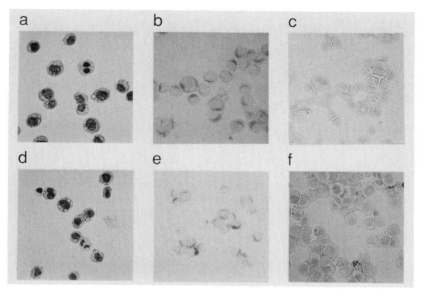

FIG. 4. Morphological and cytochemical analysis of LyD9 (a,b,c), and cocultured LyD9 cells (d,e,f). Each cells were analyzed morphology by means of May-Grünwald-Giemsa staining (a,d), and cytochemically with α-naphthyl esterase (b,e) and peroxidase (c,f). The magnification is X200. The pictures are presented from cocultured LyD9 cells with PA-6 for 4 weeks in the presence of a limited amount of IL-3.

myeloid as well as lymphoid cells in induced K-4 cells (Figure 3g and h). Furthermore, GM-CSF-dependent cell lines similar to the K-GM clone were obtained by culturing induced K-4 cells in GM-CSF. These results indicate that the K-4 clone can differentiate into myeloid cells as well as B lymphocytes when cocultured with bone marrow stroma cells. In contrast, the LS-1 and K-GM clones did not ever differentiate into B lymphocytes in the same coculture system. The results led us to conclude that the LS-1 and K-GM clones had been committed to the myeloid lineage. These results, together with the fact that the anti-IL-4 monoclonal antibody blocked the differentiation of the LyD9 clone, allowed us to conclude that the K-4 clone is an intermediate in the differentiation pathway of the LyD9 cell into myeloid cells as well as B cells.

Cloned Stroma Cell Lines Can Support Myeloid Differentiation of LyD9 Cells

We tried to replace primary bone marrow stroma cells with cloned stroma cell lines. There are two stroma lines (PA-6 and ST-2) available which are known to support myelopoiesis in the long term bone marrow culture. We found that both stroma cell lines induced LyD9 cells into myeloid cells but not B lymphocytes. Identification of myeloid cells was done by phenotypic, morphological and histochemical characterization as well as responsiveness to myeloid growth factors (GM-, M- and G-CSF). Figure 4 shows induced LyD9 cells after cultured with

PA-6 for 4 weeks. Induced LyD9 cells produced nonspecific esterase and peroxidase. Similar data were obtained with ST-2. Although ST-2 was reported to support B cell differentiation as well in the bone marrow cell culture (6), LyD9 cells were not induced to differentiate into B cells by coculture with ST-2. Failure of the B cell development with cloned stroma cell lines may be due to the suppression of lymphopoiesis by dominant myeloid cells, or requirement of different growth factors which make multipotent precursor cells to commit to B cell lineage.

DISCUSSION

Here we have demonstrated that the IL-3-dependent progenitor clone (LyD9) and its IL-4-dependent derivative (K-4) have capacities to differentiate into myeloid as well as B lymphocytes when cocultured with bone marrow stroma cells. The induced cells gave rise to long-term stroma or CSF-dependent cell clones which had differentiated into the granulocyte/macrophage lineage. Available surface markers could not distinguish between the LyD9 and K-4 clones except for the increased B220 expression on the K-4. Studies on phenotypic changes in the intermediate clone K-4 other than the growth factor requirement will provide a clue to understand molecular events required for differentiation of early precursor cells in the bone marrow.

It is interesting that IL-4 was necessary during the differentiation of LyD9 cells into B cells and granulocyte-macrophage cells since IL-4 is known to be a soluble factor which acts on T cells, B cells and mast cells (13,14). Because both multipotential K-4 cells and granulocyte-macrophage progenitor cells, LS-1 were able to respond to IL-4, IL-4 would play important roles in differentiation of hematopoietic progenitor cells in agreement with the report that IL-4 enhances the proliferation of CFU-GM, CFU-e and CFU-mix in the presence of appropriate factors (15). Although IL-4 is involved in an early phase of differentiation, IL-4 alone cannot induce differentiation of the LyD9 cell. It remains to be determined whether LyD9 cells or stroma cells produce IL-4 during the coculture. Stroma cells seem to provide differentiation signals to LyD9 and K-4 cells during their physical contact.

Several investigators (16,17) have described leukemic cells or hematopoietic cells transformed with oncogenes that express both B-cell and myeloid characters. These studies suggest the existence of a common B-cell/myeloid progenitor cell in agreement with the present study. Some other leukemic cells have properties of both the T lymphocyte and myeloid lineages. It is worth noting that both LyD9 cells (5) and HAFTL-1 cells (16) express the Ly-1 surface antigen. Ly-1$^-$ IL-3-dependent pro-B lymphocyte clones were shown to give rise *in vivo* to B lymphocytes but not to T lymphocytes or myeloid cells (3).

The second point that is clear from the present studies is that acquisition of capacities to respond to different growth factors is associated with differentiation of the LyD9 clone into B lymphocytes and myeloid cells. It will be interesting to determine whether the change of growth factor dependence is induced either by increased numbers of specific receptors or by induction of the intracellular signal transduction machinery specific to receptors. We will be able to test whether expression of a specific receptor can induce differentiation into a particular lineage when cDNAs of various receptors are available.

ACKNOWLEDGMENTS

We are grateful to Ms. J. Kuno, S. Okazaki, and K. Fujiseki for their skillful assistance and to Ms. K. Hirano for her help in preparation of the manuscript. This investigation was supported by the Ministry of Education, Culture and Science of Japan. The Basel Institute for Immunology was founded and is supported by F. Hoffmann-La Roche, Ltd. Co.

REFERENCES

1. Tonegawa, S. (1983): *Nature* 302:575-581.
2. Honjo, T., and Habu, S. (1985): *Annu. Rev. Biochem.* 54:803-830.
3. Palacios, R., and Steinmetz, M. (1985): *Cell* 41:727-734.
4. Palacios, R., and Pelkonen, J. (1988): *Immunol. Rev.* 104:1-23.
5. Palacios, R., Karasuyama, H., and Rolink, A. (1987): *EMBO J.* 6:3687-3693.
6. Ogawa, M., Nishikawa, S., Ikuta, K., Yamamura, F., Naito, M., Takahashi, K., and Nishikawa, S. I. (1988): *EMBO J.* 7:1337-1343.
7. McKearn, P. J., McCubrey, J., and Fagg, B. (1985): *Proc. Natl. Acad. Sci. USA* 82:7414-7418.
8. Kincade, P. W., Ralph, P., and Moore, M. A. S. (1976): *J. Exp. Med.* 143:1265-1270.
9. Nishikawa, S., Sasaki, Y., Kina, T., Amagai, T., and Katsura, Y. (1986): *Immunogenetics* 23:137-139.
10. Goud, Th. J. L. M., Schotte, C., and Van Furth, R. (1975): *J. Exp. Med.* 142:1180-1199.
11. Kinashi, T., Inaba, K., Tsubata, T., Tashiro, K., Palacios, R., and Honjo, T. (1988): *Proc. Natl. Acad. Sci. USA* 85:4473-4477.
12. Kinashi, T., Tashiro, K., Inaba, K., Takeda, T., Palacios, R., and Honjo, T. (1989): *Internatl. Immunol.* 1:11-19.
13. Noma, Y., Sideras, P., Naito, T., Bergstedt-Lindquist, S., Azuma, C., Severinson, E., Tanabe, T., Kinashi, T., Matsuda, F., Yaoita, Y., and Honjo, T. (1986): *Nature* 319:640-646.
14. Sideras, P., Noma, T., and Honjo, T. (1988): *Immunol. Rev.* 102:189-212.
15. Peschel, C., Paul, W. E., Ohara, J., and Green, I. (1987): *Blood* 70:254-263.
16. Davidson, F. W., Pierce, J. H., Rudikoff, S., and Morse, III, H. (1988): *J. Exp. Med.* 168:389-407.
17. Greaves, M. G., Chan, C. L., Furley, W. J. A., Watt, M. S., and Molgaard, V. H. (1986): *Blood* 67:1-11.

Molecular Aspects of Immune Response and Infectious Diseases, edited by H. Kiyono, E. Jirillo, and C. DeSimone. Raven Press, Ltd., New York, © 1990.

17

BP-1 and BP-3 Alloantigens: Cell Surface Glycoproteins Expressed by Early B Lineage Cells in Mice

K. M. McNagny*+, Q. Wu*+, P. A. Welch*+‡,
P. D. Burrows*+ and M. D. Cooper*+‡§¶

Division of Developmental and Clinical Immunology, Departments of Microbiology+, Pediatrics‡ and Medicine§, University of Alabama at Birmingham, Howard Hughes Medical Institute¶, Birmingham, Alabama 35294, USA

INTRODUCTION

Fetal liver and bone marrow provide a unique milieu for the genesis of multiple lineages of hematopoietic cells. Within these microenvironments B lymphocyte precursors undergo a sequentially ordered set of immunoglobulin gene rearrangements, polyclonal growth and differentiate into mature immunocompetent B cells (1-3). *In vitro* culture systems have demonstrated that the growth and differentiation of these B cell precursors is dependent on an adherent layer of stromal cells (4). These stromal cells are thought to be a component of what has traditionally been termed the "inductive microenvironment" which promotes B cell development *in vivo*. Although the available data indicate that both soluble factors and direct contact between pre-B and stromal cells are required for B lymphopoiesis, relatively little is known about the nature of the interactions involved in these processes at the molecular level.

In order to better characterize the molecules through which pre-B cells interact with their hemopoietic microenvironment we have used an alloimmunization strategy to produce a panel of monoclonal antibodies directed against murine pre-B cell surface antigens. Two of these antibodies, BP-1 and BP-3, recognize cell surface glycoproteins whose expression is restricted to the early stages of B cell differentiation (see Figure 1). The tissue distribution, tightly regulated expression, and biochemical properties of these two molecules suggest unique functional roles for these proteins in B lymphopoiesis.

RESULTS

In this study, a panel of murine alloantibodies was produced by hyperimmunizing *Mus spretus* wild mice with the neoplastic pre-B cell line 18.81 which is of BALB/c origin. The theory behind such an immunization strategy is that it allows the generation of antibodies against allelic forms of highly conserved proteins (5, 6). The BP-1 and BP-3 antibodies were selected from this panel for further characterization on the basis of their reactivity with subpopulations of B lineage cells and their lack of reactivity with T lineage cells (7, 8) (Table 1).

BP-1 Antigen

The antigen recognized by BP-1 is a phosphorylated cell surface glycoprotein formed by two disulfide-linked chains of 140 kDa. It is expressed on pre-B and immature B cells in hemopoietic tissues, including bone marrow, neonatal spleen, and fetal liver, as well as certain bone marrow-derived stromal cell lines (7). A different epitope of the BP-1 antigen is recognized by the rat monoclonal antibody 6C3 (9). Adkins and coworkers have shown that a subpopulation of thymic cortical epithelial cells also express the 6C3 antigen (10). Expression of the BP-1 / 6C3 antigen could not be detected on adult thymocytes, splenocytes, and cells from Peyer's patches, lymph nodes or the peritoneal cavity (7).

Because the cell surface expression of the BP-1 / 6C3 antigen is up-regulated on transformed pre-B cells and pre-B cells from Whitlock-Witte long term bone marrow cultures (9, 11-13), it has been proposed that augmented expression of this antigen might be correlated with cell transformation (9-11). However, several experimental results suggest that this is probably not the case; 1) this antigen is also expressed by cells from normal hemopoietic tissues albeit at lower levels (7, 14), and 2) the antigen is clearly absent on a number of Abelson murine leukemia virus (A-MuLV) transformed pre-B cell lines (15). However, the fact that expression of this antigen is restricted to the pre-B and very early B cell stage indicates that it is a differentiation marker and suggests it may play a role in normal B cell development (7, 14).

This possibility is further supported by analysis of *in vitro* B cell culture systems. Careful examination of Whitlock-Witte long term bone marrow cultures demonstrated that in addition to the early B lineage cells, a subpopulation of stromal cells also express the BP-1 / 6C3 antigen (16, 17). Up-regulated expression of the BP-1 / 6C3 antigen was observed on stromal cell lines that are highly supportive of pre-B cell proliferation (16, 17). When purified pre-B cells are cultured with these supportive stromal cell lines, they are induced to proliferate and rapidly increase their levels of surface BP-1 / 6C3. Similar effects could be induced when the stromal cells were replaced with stromal cell culture supernatant or with recombinant IL-7 (17, Welch, P.A. *et al.*, manuscript in preparation). The up-regulation of BP-1 / 6C3 antigen expression induced by IL-7 is highly specific. The B220 and BP-3 molecules on pre-B cells are not up-regulated and other interleukins (e.g., IL-6) fail to induce the increase in BP-1 / 6C3 expression (Welch, P.A., *et al.*, manuscript submitted). These results suggest that the BP-1 antigen may play a role in cell proliferation by acting directly as a growth factor receptor for autocrine or paracrine factors (possibly for IL-7), or indirectly by regulating the lymphokine / receptor mediated events.

To further study the structural and functional characteristics of the BP-1 / 6C3 antigen, we have cloned a cDNA encoding this molecule from a library derived from a BP-1 / 6C3+ A-MuLV transformed pre-B cell line (19). Northern blot analysis using the cDNA as a probe revealed a major 4.1 kb transcript in BP-1/6C3+ cell lines and one human pre-B cell line. The cDNA sequence predicts a 945 amino acid type II integral membrane protein that is composed of a 17 amino acid N-terminal cytoplasmic domain, a 22 amino acid membrane-spanning domain and a 906 amino acid C-terminal extracellular domain. Nine potential N-linked

TABLE 1. Characteristics of BP-1 and BP-3 antigens

Feature	BP-1	BP-3
Lymphoid distribution	μ^+ pre-B cells to immature B cells in bone marrow	μ^- B cell precursor to subpopulation of peripheral B cells
Non-lymphoid distribution	lymphopoiesis supportive stromal cells, thymic cortical epithelia, intestinal brush border, renal proximal tubule	stromal cells in peripheral lymphoid tissues, myeloid cells
Native molecular weights (core protein)	130,000 - 140,000 (110,000)	42,000 - 48,000 (32,000)
N-linked oligosaccharides	+ (nine potential sites)	+ ($\geq$ 4 sites)
Phosphorylation	+	-
Membrane anchor	type II integral membrane protein	glycosyl-phosphatidyl-inositol anchor (GPI)
Sequence homology	metallopeptidases	?

glycosylation sites, a potential sulfation site, and a typical zinc-binding motif were found in the extracellular domain. The BP-1 / 6C3 cDNA sequence shares significant amino acid sequence homology to human CD13 / aminopeptidase N (36%), and represents a second member of the zinc-dependent metallopeptidase gene family found in early B-lineage cells.

BP-3 Antigen

The antigen recognized by the BP-3 antibody exhibits a less restricted B lineage distribution than that observed for BP-1, but it also displays biochemical properties and a cell distribution pattern which suggest an important role in B cell differentiation. The BP-3 antibody recognizes a variably glycosylated cell surface protein that is expressed by all pre-B and newly formed B cells in bone marrow and by a subpopulation of B cells in peripheral lymphoid tissues (8). The majority of the BP-3[+] B cells express high levels of surface IgM, low levels of surface IgD and are relatively small in size. This immature phenotype suggests that the BP-3[+] cells in the periphery represent relatively recent emigrants from the bone marrow (19, 20), and that expression of this antigen decreases as a function of B cell maturation. A survey of neoplastic B lineage cell lines supports this conclusion as BP-3 was expressed by all pre-B cell lines at high levels and was low or absent on mature B cell lines and plasmacytomas (8).

The BP-3 antigen is not limited to the B cell lineage. Myeloid cells also express it but, in contrast to B lineage cells, the level of BP-3 expression increases as a function of myeloid cell differentiation. Myeloid cells in the bone marrow thus express relatively little antigen whereas circulating polymorphonuclear cells and peritoneal macrophages express the antigen at high levels (8).

Staining of tissue sections with the BP-3 antibody reveals a very striking spatial organization of this antigen in lymphoid organs. In the spleen, immunoreactivity is restricted to lymphoid follicles of the white pulp areas, identifying what appear to be 3-dimensional arrays or networks of stromal cells. These networks range from approximately 5 to 20 μm in diameter and form a continuous capsule around the follicles as well as an intricate intrafollicular mesh. Sequential sections stained with anti-IgD and anti-Thy-1 suggest that these arrays are most prominent within the B cell rich region of the follicles. Similar structures are detected in lymph nodes and Peyer's patches although the organization of the networks in these tissues is somewhat less well defined. Such structures are not observed in tissue sections of thymus or bone marrow suggesting that BP-3 expressing stromal cells are restricted to the peripheral lymphoid tissues. When mice are treated with sequential doses of cyclophosphamide which leads to the depletion of B and T cells a high density of BP-3 antigen is detected in the collapsed splenic follicles indicating that the residual stromal cells express the BP-3 antigen at high levels. In contrast, these BP-3[+] networks are absent in severe combined immunodeficiency (SCID) mice suggesting that lymphocytes are required for development of these organized structures.

Biochemical analysis of the BP-3 antigen revealed it to be a 32 kDa cell surface protein with at least four sites for the addition of N-linked oligosaccharides (8). Although the same 32 kDa core protein is immunoprecipitated from pre-B cell lines, bone marrow, and peritoneal macrophages, each of these tissues displays a distinct glycosylation pattern suggesting that the BP-3 antigen is post-translationally modified in a tissue and cell type-specific manner. We have recently demonstrated that treatment of both pre-B cells and peritoneal macrophages with phosphoinositide-specific phospholipase C (PI-PLC) leads to the specific release of BP-3 antigen from the cell surface suggesting that the BP-3 is anchored to the outer leaflet of the plasma membrane by a glycosyl-phosphatidylinositol (GPI) linkage (McNagny, K., unpublished observations). Molecules that share this unusual type of post-translational modification include cell surface enzymes, molecules involved in cell activation, and cell-cell or cell-matrix adhesion molecules (reviewed in 21).

DISCUSSION

The homology of BP-1 to members of the family of zinc-dependent proteases poses several interesting possibilities for its function in B cell genesis. Both CD10 / CALLA / NEP (neutral endopeptidase) and CD13 / APN (aminopeptidase N) are expressed by hemopoietic cells at specific developmental stages and by non-hemopoietic cells in a broad range of tissues, including brain, placenta, brush

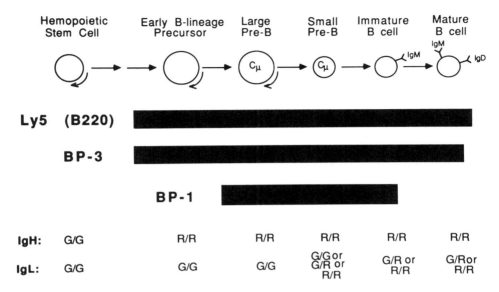

FIG. 1. Expression of B220, BP-1 and BP-3 by B lineage cells as a function of maturation. G and R indicate the configuration of the immunoglobulin gene loci: G = germline and R = rearranged.

borders of small intestines and renal proximal tubules (22, 23). Although BP-1 / 6C3 was initially identified on early B-lineage cells, the BP-1 / 6C3 antigen and mRNA expression has since been detected in liver, lungs, testis, smooth muscles, heart and brain (Wu, Q., *et al.*, unpublished observations). The detection of this ectopeptidase in such diverse tissues suggests it may have a variety of functions according to its tissue localization. It is conceivable that this molecule may play an important role in regulating cell activation or proliferation by activating or inactivating peptide hormones or interleukins.

The BP-3 molecule has not been characterized at the gene level and its role in B lymphopoiesis remains speculative. In seeking a function for this molecule it is noteworthy that many of BP-3's unique structural features have been reported for the neural cell adhesion molecule N-CAM. N-CAM is expressed by several types of neural cells and its strong homophilic nature allows cells expressing the molecule to adhere during morphogenesis (24). This molecule displays distinct differences in its glycosylation pattern between adult and embryonic tissues which fine tunes the binding affinity of the molecule during development. The embryonic form of the molecule contains an unusual polymer of sialic acid which prevents high affinity binding during the early stages of embryogenesis. The absence of this modification in adult tissue is thought to inhibit cell migration in the mature organism. In addition N-CAM is expressed by some neural cells as a GPI linked molecule (25). Although the functional significance of this modification is uncertain, this phospholipase labile anchor could provide a mechanism by which adherent cells are allowed to migrate during key stages of development.

Although the function of the BP-3 molecule remains to be elucidated, its structural and tissue distribution characteristics make it a candidate for a B cell adhesion or homing molecule. Newly formed B cells exiting the bone marrow could adhere to the BP-3$^+$ stromal cells in peripheral lymphoid organs by virtue of a homophilic interaction or by binding to another molecule expressed by these cells. Activation of phospholipases in these tissues or simply the cessation of BP-3 antigen expression following activation may provide a mechanism for the release of these cells for recirculation.

ACKNOWLEDGMENTS

The authors wish to thank Dr. J. Lahti for critical reading, and E.A. Brookshire for preparation of this manuscript.

REFERENCES

1. Cooper, M. D. (1986): In: *Progress in Immunology*, vol. VI, edited by B. Cinader, and R. G. Miller, pp. 18-32, Academic Press, New York.
2. Alt, F. W., Blackwell, T. K., DePinho, R., Reth, M., and Yancopoulos, G. (1986): *Immunol. Rev.* 89:5-30.
3. Kincade, P. W. (1987): *Adv. Immunol.* 41:181-267.
4. Whitlock, C. A., and Witte, O. N. (1982): *Proc. Natl. Acad. Sci. (USA)* 79:3608-3612.
5. Amor, M., Guenet, J., Bonhomme, F., and Cazenave, P. (1983): *Eur. J. Immunol.* 13:312-317.
6. Amor, M., Bonhomme, F., Guenet, J., Petter, F., and Cazenave, P. (1984): *Immunogenetics* 20:577-581.
7. Cooper, M. D., Mulvaney, D., Coutinho, A., and Cazenave, P. (1986): *Nature (London)* 321:616-618.
8. McNagny, K., Cazenave, P., and Cooper, M. D. (1988): *J. Immunol.* 141:2551-2556.
9. Pillemer, E., Whitlock, C. A., and Weissman, I.L. (1984): *Proc. Natl. Acad. Sci. (USA)* 82:4434-4438.
10. Adkins, B., Tidmarsh, G. F., and Weissman, I. L. (1987): *Immunogenetics* 27:180-186.
11. Tidmarsh, G. F., Dailey, M. D., and Weissman, I. L. (1986): *J. Exp. Med.* 164:1356-1361.
12. Witte, P. L., Burrows, P. D., Kincade, P. W., and Cooper, M. D. (1987): *J. Immunol.* 138:2698-2705.
13. Wu, Q., Tidmarsh, G. F., Welch, P. A., Pierce, J. H., Weissman, I. L., and Cooper, M.D. (1989): *J. Immunol.* (in press).
14. Tidmarsh, G. F., Daily, M. D., Whitlock, C. A., Pillermer, E., and Weissman, I. L. (1985): *J. Exp. Med.* 162:1421-1434.
15. Ramakrishnan, L., Wu, Q., Yue, A., Cooper, M. D., and Rosenberg, N. (1989): *J. Exp. Med.* (Submitted).
16. Whitlock, C. A., Tidmarsh, G. F., Muller-Sieburg, C., and Weissman, I. L. (1987): *Cell* 48:1009-1021.
17. Welch, P. A., Gillis, S., and Cooper, M. D. (1989): *Fed. Proc.* 3:A1271.
18. Wu, Q., Lahti, J. M., Air, G. M., Burrows, P. D., and Cooper, M. D. (1989): *Proc. Natl. Acad. Sci.* (Submitted).
19. Yuan, D., and Vitetta, E. S. (1978): *J. Immunol.* 120:353-356.
20. Abney, E. R., Hunter, I. R., and Parkhouse, R. M. E. (1976): *Nature* 259:404-406.
21. Low, M. (1989): *FASEB J.* 3:1600-1608.
22. Letarte, M., Vera, S., Tran, R., Addis, J. B. L., Onizuka, R. J., Quackenbush, E. J., Jongeneel, C. V., and Mcinnes, R. R. (1988): *J. Exp. Med.* 168:1247-1253.
23. Look, A. T., Ashmun, R. A., Shapiro, L. H., and Peiper, S. C. (1989): *J. Clin. Invest.* 83:1299-1307.

24. Edelman, G. M. (1985): *Annu. Rev. Biochem.* 54:135-169.
25. He, H., Barbet, J., Chaix, J., and Goridis, C. (1986): *EMBO* 5:2489-2494.

Molecular Aspects of Immune Response and Infectious Diseases, edited by H. Kiyono, E. Jirillo, and C. DeSimone. Raven Press, Ltd., New York, © 1990.

18

Principles of B Cell Selection *In Vivo*

K. Rajewsky

Institute for Genetics, University of Cologne, Weyertal 121, D-5000 Cologne 41, Federal Republic of Germany

The somatic evolution of the antibody repertoire in the mouse proceeds through clonal expansion and selection of B cells. These processes can be studied through the molecular analysis of antibody V regions expressed by B cells in various compartments of the immune system, combined with the determination of their proliferation dynamics at various stages of development. For the latter purpose we use a technique which involves labeling of the cells with 5-bromo-deoxyuridine in vivo and subsequent multiparameter flow cytometric analysis of the labeled cells (1).

Two basic pathways of B cell differentiation emerge. In the first, long-lived B cells, many of which carry the Ly1 marker, are generated early in life (2). In the adult mouse these B cells show little proliferative activity. However, the molecular analysis of their antibody V regions indicates strong clonal expansion and selection of particular sets of V regions, in the absence of somatic mutation (3). Occasionally, these processes result in the development of chronic B cell leukemia. The expansion of a selected, germ line encoded antibody repertoire in this compartment meets the requirements of "natural" immunity (4).

In the second B cell differentiation pathway, that of acquired immunity, antigen-induced somatic "memory" is gene-rated (4-6). Here, stepwise intraclonal maturation of antibody affinity occurs through V region hypermutation and cellular selection in the course of clonal expansion (7). This expansion starts either from B cells newly generated from stem cells in the bone marrow, or from a population of stable B cells selected from the former into the peripheral B cell pool (8). T cell help is required for the induction of B cell memory; less, if any, help is needed for its maintenance which may thus be based on long-lived memory cells (9; P. Vieira and K. Rajewsky, submitted for publication). In the effector phases of acquired B cell immunity, the 1º and 2º antibody response, hypermutation does not occur and a stable antibody repertoire is expressed (10).

ACKNOWLEDGEMENTS

The work from my laboratory quoted in this article was supported by the Deutsche Forschungsgemeinschaft through SFBs 74 and 243 and by the Fazit Foundation.

REFERENCES

1. Förster, I., Vieira, P., and Rajewsky, K. (1989): *Int. Immunol.* 1:321-331.
2. Herzenberg, L. A., Stall, A. M., Lalor, P. A., Sidman, C., Moore, W. A., Parks, D. R., and Herzenberg, L. A. (1986): *Immunol. Rev.* 93:81-102.
3. Förster, I., Gu, H., and Rajewsky, K. (1988): *EMBO J.* 7:3693-3703.
4. Rajewsky, K., Förster, I., and Cumano, A. (1987): *Science* 238:1088-1094.
5. Berek, C., and Milstein, C. (1988): *Immunol. Rev.* 105:1-26.
6. Kocks, C., and Rajewsky, K. (1989): *Ann. Rev. Immunol.* 7:537-559.
7. Kocks, C., and Rajewsky, K. (1988): *Proc. Natl. Acad. Sci. USA* 85:8206-8210.
8. Rajewsky, K. (1989): In *Cold Spring Harbor Symp. Quant. Biol.*, Cold Spring Harbor.
9. Rajewsky, K. (1989): In *Progress in Immunology*, vol. VII, edited by Melchers, F., *et al.*, pp. 397-403, Springer-Verlag, Heidelberg.
10. Siekevitz, M., Kocks, C., Rajewsky, K., and Dildrop, R. (1987): *Cell* 48:757-770.

Molecular Aspects of Immune Response and Infectious Diseases, edited by H. Kiyono, E. Jirillo, and C. DeSimone. Raven Press, Ltd., New York, © 1990.

19

Hemopoietic Stem Cells and Early Hematolymphoid Differentiation in Mouse / Man

I. Weissman, S. Heimfeld, G. Spangrude, R. Namikawa, M. Lieberman, H. Kaneshima, L. Smith, C. Guidos, B. Adkins, and M. McCune

Stanford University School of Medicine, Stanford, California 94305, USA

The study of mammalian hematolymphopoiesis offers to the developmental biologist at the same time a system that allows precise analysis of *in vitro* models and *in vivo* outcomes, as well as the possibility of rapid transfer of obtained knowledge to contemporary clinical problems. Using antibodies directed against hematolymphoid lineage markers with various cell-sorting strategies for the adoptive transfer of cells between congenic mouse strains we have recently isolated 1) the pluripotent hematopoietic stem cell; 2) a multipotent progenitor that apparently does not self renew; and 3) several lineage specific progenitors (Table 1).

Using a similar technology, we have isolated three classes of intrathymic T cell progenitors, as assayed by intrathymic transfer of cells into the thymus of unirradiated cogenic hosts (Table 2).

In order to study parallel developmental processes in human hematolymphoid differentiation, and especially, to provide models to study the pathogenesis of human hematotropic and lymphotropic viruses (such as HIV), we have established a working model of human lymphopoiesis in immunodeficient (SCID) mice. Implantation of human fetal thymus under the SCID mouse kidney capsule allows full development of thymocytes and peripheral T cells from i.v. injected human fetal liver hematopoietic cells. Implantation of human fetal lymph nodes (and/or spleen) allows reconstitution of lymphoid cells. Preliminary studies indicate that these hosts will prove useful in the identification of human hematolymphoid progenitors, and to study the *in vivo* pathogenetic potential of molecularly cloned HIV.

TABLE 1. Mouse hematopoietic progenitor cells

Cell Name	Cell-Surface Phenotype	Developmental Outcome	Comments
Hematopoietic Stem Cell	Thy-1^{lo} Lin$^-$ Scal$^-$	Self-Renewal all hemat. progeny	App. homog.; 30 cells save 50% of LIH
Multipotent heterogen. Progenitors	Thy-1^{lo} M$^+$G$^+$B$^+$ Scal$^+$	No self-renewal All hematolymp. progeny	Poss. will not save LIH
Myelomonocitic Progenitor	Thy-1^{lo} M$^+$G$^+$B$^-$ Scal$^-$	Monocytes Macrophages Granulocytes	8-day CFU-S
Pre-B Progenitor	Thy-1^{lo} M$^-$G$^-$B$^+$ Scal$^-$	B lineage only	Efficient Ab-MuLV target

TABLE 2. Mouse hematopoietic progenitor cells

Progenitor Group	Cell-Surface Phenotype	Developmental Outcome	Comments
1	Thy-1^{hi} CD4$^-$, CD8$^-$ TCR$^-$	All thymic and T cells	Extensive but non unlimited self-renewal;
2	Thy-1^{hi} CD4$^-$, CD8$^+$ TCR$^-$	Non mature and mature thymocytes T cells	Derived from progenitor 1; gives rise to progenitor 3;
3	Thy-1^{hi} CD4$^+$, CD8$^+$ TCR$^-$	Non mature and mature thymocytes T cells	Derived from progenitor 2[a]

[a]Immediate progeny begin to express low levels of TCR.

Molecular Aspects of Immune Response and Infectious
Diseases, edited by H. Kiyono, E. Jirillo, and
C. DeSimone. Raven Press, Ltd., New York, © 1990.

20

Implications of Idiotypes in Infectious Diseases and Other Pathological Conditions

K. Eichmann

Max-Planck-Institut für Immunbiologie, Freiburg, Federal Republic of Germany

HISTORICAL BACKGROUND

When myeloma proteins, the unusual "paraproteins" of patients with multiple myeloma, where first suspected to be related to normal immunoglobulins, one way of testing this relationship was to produce antisera to myeloma proteins and to study their crossreactivity with normal γ-globulin preparations. In 1953, Lohss *et al.* reported that "in two out of three antisera to myeloma-γ-globulin fractions a small proportion of remaining antibodies were demonstrated which could be saturated neither with normal γ-globulin nor with total serum" (1). This was a first description of anti-idiotypic antibodies, i.e., antibodies that recognize unique (ιδιοσ = peculiar, distinct) features of a homogeneous immunoglobulin or antibody molecule that do not appear to be associated with normal, heterogeneous immunoglobulins or with other homogeneous immunoglobulins. In the following years, the major contributions to the understanding of the phenomenon were made by the laboratories of Oudin (2) and of Kunkel (3). Even from this early work it became clear that the "idiotype" of a homogeneous antibody or myeloma protein was the serological reflection of its unique structure in the variable domain. Due to the enormous diversity of normal immunoglobulins, molecules with an idiotype similar to that of any given individual immunoglobulin molecule usually remain below the level of detection.

BASIC CONCEPTS OF IDIOTYPES

Structural Considerations

Immunoglobulin (Ig) molecules are composed of heavy and light polypeptide chains. Each of these polypeptide chains consists of a variable and constant portion. Whereas the amino acid sequences of the variable portions are unique to individual antibody molecules, the amino acid sequences of the constant portions are invariant within one class or type of antibody heavy and light chains. The variable and constant regions of both heavy and light chains are folded according to β sheet structure, and two double layer β sheets, one contributed by the heavy chain variable region and the other by the light chain variable region, together form the variable (V) domain of an immunoglobulin molecule (4). The amino acid sequence variability in Ig variable regions is not randomly distributed but accumulates in 3 hypervariable complementarity determining regions interspaced by less variable frame-work regions (5). Due to the folding of the molecule, 3 heavy chain and 3 light chain complementarity determining regions become exposed towards the outer surface of the V domain to form the continuous surface of a cleft of varying shape and depth, the antigen-binding site (4, 5).

Although a direct biophysical demonstration is still missing, there is no doubt that the antigen-binding site of an antibody molecule contributes to or determines its idiotype (reviewed in 6). This is most directly shown by a host of experiments in which competition between the binding of antigen and the binding of anti-idiotypic antibodies to an antibody was demonstrated. By such techniques interaction sites for monoclonal anti-idiotypic antibodies (idiotopes) have been located in most cases as partially overlapping with the antigen binding site, rarely as virtually identical with it. Additional approaches to relate idiotypes to structural features of Ig molecules included the sequence analysis of structurally closely related Ig molecules such as somatic point mutants. These experiments demonstrated that idiotopes are sensitive to small structural variations, mostly within hypervariable sequence regions but in some cases also to those in framework regions (reviewed in 6). A final understanding of the molecular events taking place upon the idiotypic interaction of two antibody molecules will have to await the cocrystallisation of such complexes and their analysis by X-ray crystallography.

Idiotypic Cross-Specificity; Major Idiotypes

Whereas in the initial studies on idiotypes the astonishing specificity for individual antibody molecules ("individual antigen specificity") was in the center of attention, it became obvious later that antibody molecules of different origin may share idiotypic properties, i.e., react with the same anti-idiotypic antibody. This was first noted in studies on the genetic control of antibody responses, in which it was shown that different members of families of rabbits or of inbred strains of mice, when immunized with certain antigens, produced antibodies with similar or related idiotypes (reviewed in 7, 8). Such idiotypes, associated with antibodies predictably induced by a defined antigen in a genetically defined situation, were termed "major idiotypes." The existence of major idiotypes gave rise to a host of studies to evaluate their possible immunoregulatory function, or their suitability as targets for immunomanipulation (reviewed in 9, 10). These studies are now historical but layed the ground for present day considerations on idiotypes in the interpretation of various medical conditions or on the use of anti-idiotypic antibodies for medical manipulations (see below).

The Notion of Internal Image

Complementary shapes of the surfaces of antibody combining sites and antigen are prerequisites for specific antigen-antibody binding. Similarly, anti-idiotypic antibodies must have binding sites complementary to regions associated with the binding sites of another antibody. In some extreme cases, indirect but compelling evidence leads to the conclusion that the binding sites of two antibodies can be essentially complementary to one another. In such cases, the combining site of one of the antibodies is an exact image of the antigen, i.e., the epitope for which the other antibody is specific. Hence, external antigens may have "internal images" in the immune system. As mentioned above, the experimental evidence leading to these conclusions is indirect and based on observations on anti-idiotypic antibodies that react with virtually all antibodies, even those derived from different species, against a given antigen. For binding to an anti-idiotypic antibody that represents an internal image of the antigen, there is no requirement for structural similarity that would go beyond the similarity required for antibodies to be reactive with the same epitope.

The Network Theory

Combining the above considerations with the knowledge on the enormous diversity of the antibody system and on the degeneracy of antigen-antibody interactions, Jerne proposed that most if not all antibody molecules would find at least a few complementary antibody molecules within the same individual. While many of these complementary antibodies would be anti-idiotypic in a normal sense, some others would be internal images of external antigens. If this was indeed the case, there would be numerous idiotypic interactions going on at any one time in the immune system. Moreover, the reaction of the immune system to an antigen would involve not only those antibodies which are complementary to the antigen but also further antibodies that are complementary to the initial antibodies. Hence, networks of spreading reactions would occur among complementary sets of antibodies: Ab_1 ... Ab_2 ... Ab_3 etc. each consisting of ordinary anti-idiotypes (α set) and internal image like anti-idiotypes (β set). The β sets of all odd numbered Ab's would be reactive with the antigen whereas the β sets of even numbered Ab's would be internal images of the antigen. Jerne further proposed that these spreading reactions, particularly through the α sets, have regulatory, i.e., enhancing or suppressive consequences for the immune response. Moreover, he proposed that network interactions in general would be important to maintain steady states in the immune system (11, 12).

The network theory has remained a controversial subject. While idiotypic complementarities among antibodies within the immune system have been demonstrated in many instances, their exact functional consequences have remained elusive. Nevertheless, the network theory has formed the theoretical framework for experimentation on artificial manipulation of the immune system by administration of anti-idiotypic antibodies, now being considered to be of possible use for certain medical problems (see below).

Idiotypes of T Cell Antigen Receptors

The MHC restricted, antigen-specific reactivity of T lymphocytes is conferred by a molecular complex consisting of 5 invariant transmembrane polypeptides, together termed CD3, and the $\alpha\beta$ heterodimer, two polypeptide chains consisting of variable and constant portions similar to but not identical with immunoglobulin molecules (reviewed in 13, 14, 15). While it is not known in detail how this molecule binds to the MHC/antigen complex, DNA transfection experiments have unequivocally assigned the MHC/antigen specificity to the $\alpha\beta$ heterodimer (14).

The diversity of this receptor system is potentially of similar magnitude as that of antibodies (reviewed in 15).

The discovery of the molecular identity of the T cell receptor in the early 1980's involved the use of anti-idiotypic antibodies (13, 16). These were made by injecting whole *in vitro* cloned T cells, thus obtaining monoclonal antibodies that reacted only with the injected T cell clone and not with others. The resulting "anti-clonotypic" antibodies were then shown to bind to a heterodimeric membrane protein on the T cell surface which was later demonstrated to confer specific recognition. While these and subsequent studies showed that T cell receptors bear idiotypic properties, little is known to date about the physiological role of such idiotypes, or their potential as targets for immunomanipulation.

Manipulation of Immune Responses by Anti-Idiotypic Antibodies

Heart *et al.* were the first to demonstrate that injection of anti-idiotypic antibodies into mice resulted in the elimination of idiotype-bearing antibodies from the subsequent immune response to the antigen (17). In later work, several other groups have investigated the details of idiotype suppression, leading to the definition of two essentially different forms of the phenomenon: a short term suppression with rapid recovery and a long term suppression that is maintained by an active process in the animal. The dose of anti-idiotype injected and the age of the animal determine which form of suppression is induced (reviewed in 9, 10).

The initial demonstration that anti-idiotypic antibodies could also serve as inducers of immunity was made in the immune responses to a bacterial polysaccharide. Mice of strain A/J, when immunized with Group A streptococci, made antibodies to the cell wall polysaccharide of these bacteria that carried a major idiotype. Anti-idiotypic antibodies to this idiotype, when injected into naive A/J mice, primed these mice to mount a secondary immune response when challenged later with the bacteria (reviewed in 9). Induction of specific immune responses by anti-idiotypic antibodies was subsequentially demonstrated in a number of other experimental systems (reviewed in 9, 10, 18). Whereas low doses of anti-idiotypic antibodies induced the immune response or primed the animal, high doses were shown to be suppressive (9, 10).

ROLE OF IDIOTYPES IN PATHOLOGICAL CONDITIONS

Idiotypic Vaccination

The concept of the internal image, together with the observations on induction of immunity by anti-idiotypic antibodies gave rise to considerations towards the use of anti-idiotypic antibodies as vaccines. In the following years numerous groups have performed experiments in which induction of protective immunity to several bacteria, viruses, and parasites was achieved by treating experimental animals with anti-idiotypic antibodies (Table 1) (reviewed in 18-22).

In order to study whether the basic rules of idiotypic manipulation apply in humans as well as in animals, Emmrich and collaborators studied the idiotypic properties of the human immune response to group A streptococci (reviewed in 18). While most previous work on human idiotypes had dealt with myeloma proteins or natural antibodies, these studies demonstrated the existence of major idiotypes and of internal image like anti-idiotypes, for a human anti-bacterial antibody response. Moreover, it could be demonstrated that human B cells can be

TABLE 1. Anti-idiotypic vaccinations in experimental animals[a]

Organism	Host
Virus:	
Rheovirus type 3	Mouse
Hepatitis B	Mouse, Chimpanzee
Rabies	Mouse
Poliovirus type II	Mouse
Sendai virus	Mouse
Venezuelian equine encephalomyelitis virus	Mouse
Herpes simplex virus	
Parasites:	
Trypanosoma rhodesiense	Mouse
Trypanosoma cruzi	Mouse
Shistosoma mansoni	Rat
Bacteria:	
Escherichia coli	Mouse
Streptococcus pneumoniae	Mouse
Listeria monocytogenes	Mouse

[a]Reviewed in 18-22.

induced by anti-idiotypic antibodies to secrete antibodies specific to the antigen (23).

However, considerations as to the necessity or purpose of human idiotypic vaccination may limit the applicability of this approach to cases in which alternative procedures, such as recombinant vaccines, have little chance of success (18). One such case is the problem of infant meningitis. Infants develop this disease because they fail to make antibodies to the capsular polysaccharides of the causative agents, Neisseria meningitidis or streptococcus Group B. In experimental animals it could be shown that even though newborns failed to respond to bacterial polysaccharides, they could effectively produce such antibodies if pretreated with appropriate anti-idiotypic antibodies (24). Because polysaccharides appear to be ineffective as vaccines in newborn individuals, anti-idiotypes may be considered as a useful alternative.

Idiotypes in Anti-Tumor Treatment

Anti-idiotypic antibodies have been used to treat patients with B lymphoma or chronic lymphocytic leukemia, tumors that carry monoclonal Ig as surface molecules and thus display idiotypes as cell associated tumor antigens. While in a few cases remissions were reported, these seem to be rather the exception. Lack of success in most attempts may have a number of reasons including the modulation or mutation of surface immunoglobulin of the tumor cells (reviewed in 25). No reports are available on the treatment of T cell leukemia with antibodies to clonotypic structures.

Idiotypes have also been implicated in the successful treatment of patients with colorectal cancer using monoclonal antibodies to a common antigen on these tumors. Anti-idiotype responses to the injected antibody were observed in the patients and the details of the achieved remissions were interpreted to suggest an important role of the anti-idiotype in the remission process (reviewed in 25). The concept behind this interpretation is based on the notion of internal image, such that the induced anti-idiotypic response would include antibodies that represent internal images of the cancer antigen. These internal image antibodies would then be more effective than the cancer antigen in inducing or maintaining effective anti-cancer immunity. While these interpretations have thus far remained at the level of speculation, the clinical observations certainly warrant further investigation and may give rise to useful anti-cancer treatment regimes.

Idiotypic Aspects of Autoantibodies and Other Pathogenic Antibodies

Pathogenic antibody responses occur in a variety of clinical conditions. For example various forms of allergy are caused by antibodies of IgE class, which bind to mast cells in the tissues and, upon combining with the allergen, cause mediator release from the mast cells leading to allergic symptoms (25). Pathogenic antibodies occur in a number of diseases with autoimmune ethiopathogenesis, such as rheumatoid arthritis, lupus erythematosus, myastenia gravis, autoimmune thyroiditis, etc. (reviewed in 25, 26). In the cases of anti-Ig autoantibodies ("rheumatoid factors") or anti-DNA antibodies in lupus erythematosus, it has been shown that they carry major, crossreactive idiotypes (27, 28), thus opening the possibility for suppression procedures using anti-idiotypic antibodies. Serious attempts to do so, however, have not been undertaken.

Diseases such as diabetes or hemophilia may be caused or aggravated by antibodies to insulin or factor VIII, which inactivate these mediators or cause resistance to substitution therapy. In such cases, spontaneous anti-idiotype

TABLE 2. Biological ligand-receptor systems in which molecular mimicry by anti-idiotypic antibodies has been demonstrated[a]

Hormones:
Insulin
Thyroid stimulating hormone
Prolactin
Glucogone
Vasopressin
Glucocorticoids
Neurotransmitters:
Acetylcholine
Endorphins
Catecholamines
Dopamine
Retinol binding protein
Virus:
Reovirus
Murine Leucemia virus

[a]Reviewed in 26,32.

production has been observed, together with improvement of the condition or with the loss of resistance to the therapy (29). Moreover, it has in some cases proven helpful to infuse patients with pools of heterogeneous immunoglobulin. While the reasons for the beneficial effects are not thoroughly understood, there is good reasons to suspect that idiotypic recognition between the unwanted antibodies and antibodies within the injected pool may play a role. Studies have been performed that demonstrate the spontaneous occurrence of idiotypic complexes within pools of heterogeneous immunoglobulin (30). It can, therefore, readily be imagined that an additional antibody population to be exposed to the pool may undergo complex formation with pool-derived antibodies and may thus became neutralized. Such a mechanism may account for the neutralizing effect of pooled immunoglobulin towards unwanted antibodies circulating in patients.

In studying antibodies to insulin-receptor, Sege and Peterson were the first to demonstrate that anti-idiotypic antibodies (Ab_2) could be perfect images of the antigen reactive with Ab_1 (31). Moreover, they showed for the case of insulin receptor that such internal image antibodies could functionally replace the hormone in hormone-receptor interactions leading to cell signalling. In the following years, similar results were reported for several other hormone-receptor systems (reviewed in 25, 26, 32). Together, these studies demonstrated that anti-idiotypic antibodies have the general capacity to mimick non-immunoglobulin structures, be they hormone receptors or other molecules (Table 2). Molecules mimicked by anti-idiotypic antibodies have in most cases been proteins, but evidence exists that, at least in an operational sense, this may also be the case for carbohydrate antigens and other molecules (9, 10, 18, 19). Molecular mimicry of hormone receptors or other self molecules have been implicated in the ethiopathogenesis of a number of autoimmune diseases. These implications have been fostered by the numerous reports on spontaneous anti-idiotypic antibodies in a number of autoimmune and other diseases (Table 3). They may influence the course of the disease in various ways, for example by the formation of immune complexes, the consumption of complement, or by enhancement or suppression of the autoimmune process (reviewed in 26).

TABLE 3. Spontaneous anti-idiotypes in autoimmune diseases and other conditions[a]

Condition	Antigen
Cryoglobulineamia	unknown
Rheumatoid arthritis	unknown
Myastenia gravis	acetylcholin receptor
Diabetes	Insulin receptor
Systemic lupus erythematosus	DNA
Hepatitis	Hepatocyte lipoprotein
B cell lymphoma	Idiotype of lymphoma
IgA deficiency	Casein
Tetanus vaccination	Tetanus toxoid
Pregnancy	Paternal HLA
Rye sensitivity	Rye I

[a]Reviewed in 25, 26, 27, 28.

A highly interesting implication of molecular mimicry is recently discussed in connection with a possible management of AIDS. Based on the function of the T cell marker CD4 as the receptor for HIV, several groups have produced anti-idiotypic antibodies to anti-CD4 antibodies with a view to produce internal images of the CD4 binding site for HIV. Such antibodies have indeed been generated as demonstrated by their ability to bind to the GP120 envelope protein that carries the interaction site for CD4 (33). The existence of such antibodies and their ability to neutralize HIV infectivity (33) have fostered ideas on the possible induction of such antibodies by special vaccination procedures in man.

Taken together, the phenomenon of idiotypy and its many implications have deeply penetrated current concepts on ethiopathogenesis and prospective planning for future management of a variety of disease conditions. While many of these ideas are certainly bound to remain inapplicable, the intense research on idiotypes in the past and present will have been worth its while if only one of them can be developed towards a beneficial use.

SUMMARY

Idiotypes are antigenic determinants (epitopes) on antigen-specific immunological receptor molecules, including antibodies and T cell receptors. Idiotypic epitopes are associated with the antigen-combining site of these receptor molecules, resulting in a vast idiotypic heterogeneity reflecting the structural heterogeneity of antibodies and T cell receptors. Anti-idiotypic antibodies, conventional and monoclonal, can be used to manipulate the immune system, i.e., to either induce or suppress immune responses. Moreover, it has been suggested that idiotypic interactions are essential in the immune system whose function is dependent on the formation of networks of interacting molecules and cells. Idiotypes are being considered to be of importance in 3 areas of human medicine. 1. The observations that anti-idiotypic antibodies can be used to induce or enhance immune responses have fostered considerations on their possible use as vaccines for the prevention of infectious diseases. 2. Anti-idiotypic antibodies are induced in patients as a result of the therapy of cancer and other diseases with monoclonal antibodies. They may positively or negatively influence the success of these therapeutic measures. 3. Spontaneous anti-idiotypic antibodies to autoantibodies and to other pathogenic antibodies are observed in autoimmune diseases and other pathological conditions. Such anti-idiotypic antibodies have been shown to modify the course of disease. As a result of these observations, idiotypes are considered to be of interest in the ethiopathogenesis of human disease and as potential targets for human immunomanipulation.

REFERENCES

1. Lohss, F., Weiler, E., Hillman, G. (1953): *Z. Naturforsch.* 8:625-631.
2. Oudin, J., Michel, M. (1963): *C.R. Acad Sci. (Paris)* 275:805-808.
3. Kunkel, H. G. (1965): *Harvey Lect.* 59:219-232.
4. Marquart, M., and Deisenhofer, J. (1983): *Immunol. Today* 3:160-166.
5. Kabat, F. A. (1978): *Adv. Prot. Chem.* 32:1-25.
6. Kabat, F. A. (1984): In: *The Biology of Idiotypes*, edited by M. I. Greene, and A. Nissonoff, pp. 3-18, Plenum Press, New York.
7. Eichmann, K. (1975): *Immunogenetics* 2:491-527.
8. Weigert, M., and Riblet, R. (1978): *Springer's Sem. Immunopathol.* 1:133-169.

9.   Eichmann, K. (1978): *Adv. Immunol.* 26:195-254.
10. Rajewsky, K., and Takemori, T. (1983): *Ann. Rev. Immunol.* 1:569-607.
11. Jerne, N. K. (1974): *Ann. Immunol. (Int. Pasteur)* 125C:373-381.
12. Jerne, N. K. (1975): *Harvey Lect.* 70:93-111.
13. Marrack, P., and Kappler, J. (1986): *Adv. Immunol.* 38:1-39.
14. Dembic, Z. V., Boehmer, H., and Steinmetz, M. (1986): *Immunol. Today* 7:308-311.
15. Kronenberg, M., Siu, G., Hood, L., and Shastri, N. (1986): *Ann. Rev. Immunol.* 4:529-562.
16. Meuer, S. C., Fitzgerald, K. A., Hussey, K. E., Hodgon, J. C., Schlossman, S. F., and Reinherz, E. L. (1983): *J. Exp. Med.* 157:705-717.
17. Hart, D. A., Wang, A. L., Pawlak, L. L., and Nisonoff, A. (1972): *J. Exp. Med.* 135:1293-1300.
18. Eichmann, K., Emmrich, F., and Kaufmann, S. H. E. (1987): *CRC Crit. Rev. Immunol.* 7:193-227.
19. Zanetti, M., Sercarz, E., and Salk, J. (1987): *Immunol. Today* 8:18-25.
20. Bona, C. A. (1987): *La Recherche* 18:672-682.
21. Kennedy, R. C., Melnik, J. L., and Dreesman, G. K. (1986): *Sci. Am.* 255:40-48.
22. Kleber-Emmons, T., Ward, K. E., Raychaudhuri, S., Rein, R., and Köhler, H. (1986): *Int. Rev. Immunol.* 1:1-34.
23. Bloem, A., Zenke, G., Eichmann, K., and Emmrich, F. (1988): *J. Immunol.* 140:277-282.
24. Stein, K. E., and Söderström, T. (1984): *J. Exp. Med.* 160:1001-1010.
25. Geha, R. S. (1986): *Adv. Immunol.* 39:255-297.
26. Burdette, S., and Schwartz, R. S. (1987): *New Engl. J. Med.* 317:219-224.
27. Chen, P. P., Fong, S., and Carson, D. A. (1987): *Rheumatic Disease Clinics of North America* 13:545-568.
28. Pisetsky, D. S. (1987): *Rheumatic Disease Clinics of North America* 13:569-592.
29. Sultan, Y., Rossi, F., and Kazatchkine, M. D. (1987): *Proc. Natl. Acad. Sci. (USA)* 84:823-831.
30. Gronski, P., Bauer, R., Bodenbender, L., Boland, P., Diderrich, G., Hartus, H. -G., Kanzy, E. J., Kühn, K., Schmidt, K. H., Walter, G., Wiedemann, H., Zilg, H., and Seiler, S. R. (1988): *Behring Inst. Mitt.* 82:144-153.
31. Sege, K., and Peterson, P. A. (1978): *Proc. Natl. Acad. Sci. (USA)* 75:2443-2447.
32. Farid, N. R., and Lo, T. C. Y. (1985): *Endocr. Rev.* 6:1-23.
33. Dalgleish, A. G., Thomson, B. J., Chauh, T. C., Malkowski, M., and Kennedy, R. C. (1987): *Lancet* 7:1047-1049.

Molecular Aspects of Immune Response and Infectious Diseases, edited by H. Kiyono, E. Jirillo, and C. DeSimone. Raven Press, Ltd., New York, © 1990.

21

Progress Toward Vaccine Against Schistosomiasis

A. Capron, J. M. Balloul, D. Grezel, J. M. Grzych, I. Wolowczuk, C. Auriault, D. Boulanger, M. Capron, and R. J. Pierce.

Centre d'Immunologie et de Biologie Parasitaire, Unité Mixte INSERM U 167 - CNRS 624, Institut Pasteur, 1 rue du Prof. Calmette, 59019 LILLE Cédex, France

INTRODUCTION

Schistosomiasis is a chronic, debilitating disease that affects over 200 million people worldwide, and of which around 800,000 die annually according to WHO estimates. Three species of schistosome infect man (*Schistosoma mansoni*, *S. haematobium* and *S. japonicum*) while a fourth species (*S. bovis*) infects cattle, causing extensive economic loss, particularly in East Africa. Despite the existence of effective chemotherapeutic agents, and numerous programs aimed at controlling the fresh water snail intermediate host, progress towards circumscribing the parasite has been slow. This may in part due to inadequate planning of chemotherapy campaigns (1). However, the problem of drug resistance (2) and the overall economic cost mean that other approaches are necessary. Since, unlike protozoan parasites, schistosomes do not replicate in the definitive vertebrate hosts, a partial non-sterilizing immunity would greatly diminish both transmission levels in endemic areas, and the incidence of human pathology caused by the deposition of parasite eggs in host tissues (3).

An effective vaccine would reduce individual worm burdens (but not completely prevent infection) and possibly affect the fecundity of female worms. In addition, a direct effect on eggs and on egg-induced granuloma formation may be possible. All three of these effects would lead to reduced levels of pathology and diminish transmission.

The detailed knowledge that has accumulated concerning immunity to schistosomiasis, and of the target molecules of acquired immunity has meant that a number of the latter have been identified and cloned (4). This paper will outline the approaches we have undertaken towards the characterization and cloning of protective antigens, and the prospects for a viable vaccine in the light of our increasing knowledge of the immune response to the recombinant antigens.

PROTECTIVE IMMUNITY AGAINST SCHISTOSOMES

Differences in mechanisms of protective immunity are evident between experimental models and the mechanisms operating in man are as yet unknown although common characteristics exist between rat and human responses.

Mice develop immunity to reinfection after vaccination with irradiated cercariae and this resistance is T cell dependent in vivo (5). Vaccinated mice produce activated, larvicidal macrophages at the site of challenge infection. In vitro studies indicate that T lymphocytes activated by schistosome antigens produce lymphokines including gamma interferon (IFNγ) capable of activating macrophages to kill newly transformed larvae or 2 1/2 week old schistosomes (6). However, antibodies and other cell types may be involved in immunity. Murine monoclonal antibodies with specificity for schistosomulum surface antigens can mediate protection (7). Furthermore, a mechanism whereby eosinophils are responsible for very early attrition of the infection in the skin of CBA/Ca mice has been proposed (8). Most data indicate that 'late' immunity acting when schistosomula migrate from the lungs to the hepatic portal system is dominant in the mouse model (9).

The rat is a semi-permissive host developing a strong antibody-dependent immunity that is characterized by a marked anaphylactic antibody response, and the presence of antibody-dependent cellular cytotoxicity mechanisms (ADCC). The latter involve anaphylactic antibody isotypes and eosinophils, macrophages or platelets (10). These mechanisms can also operate in vivo as is suggested by the fact that the passive transfer of any of the three cell types from an infected rat will protect a naive animal against infection (11, 12). Equally, monoclonal antibodies of both rat anaphylactic antibody classes (IgG2a and IgE) have been produced that protect rats by passive transfer (13, 14).

The same in vitro effector mechanisms can be demonstrated using human or primate infection sera and cells (10) and the human immune response is also characterized by the production of high levels of anaphylactic antibodies. A further correlate to the rat model is the production of blocking antibodies recognizing schistosomulum surface carbohydrate epitopes (15), the presence of which is associated with a state of susceptibility to reinfection in human populations (16).

In practical terms, both investigations of the target antigens of immunity in the mouse model in which cell-mediated responses were studied, and the characterization of antigens responsible for humoral responses, and that were targets of ADCC mechanisms, have led to the cloning of proteins that protect against infection. The main thrust of current work in this area is directed at elucidating the types of immune responses that these molecules elicit in primates and humans (4).

TARGET ANTIGENS OF IMMUNITY

Schistosomulum surface antigens

The search for target antigens of the immune response that would be good candidate vaccine molecules first focused on those determinants expressed on the surface of the schistosomulum. Newly transformed schistosomula have a restricted repertoire of molecules at their surface (17) of which the immunodominant species is a 38 kD glycoprotein (GP38). This molecule was first identified (18) using a rat monoclonal IgG2a antibody (IPLSm1) that mediated both eosinophil-dependent cytotoxicity towards schistosomula and protection of rats by passive transfer (19). Subsequent studies have shown that the epitope involved in the protective response was glycannic in nature (20). This, taken together with the fact that the antibody response to GP38 produced both protective (IgG2a) and blocking (IgG2c) subclasses in rats (19) and the existence of such blocking antibodies (of the IgM class) in human sera (15) meant that the molecular cloning of the protein portion of GP38 would be both difficult and of limited usefulness.

For this reason, an anti-idiotype strategy was developed, based on the IPLSm1 antibody (21). Rats immunized with a monoclonal anti-idiotype antibody (AB2) directed against the antigen-binding site of IPLSm1 produced specific AB3 antibodies that were highly cytotoxic for schistosomula in vitro in the presence of eosinophils, and protected rats against infection by passive transfer. Equally, immunization of rats with AB2 antibodies protected rats against infection.

At this stage, the characterization of the glycan epitope was facilitated by a chance observation when using keyhole limpet hemocyanin (KLH) as a carrier for the immunization of rats with the AB2 monoclonal antibody, that control animals immunized with KLH alone developed antibodies to GP38 (22). This result tallied with parallel work showing that the glycan epitope of GP38 was shared not only with the intermediate host of *S. mansoni*, *Biomphalaria glabrata*, but with other fresh water snails including schistosome hosts such as *Bulinus truncatus* and non-hosts such as *Limnaea limosa* (23).

The availability of KLH has meant that structural analysis of the glycans reaching with IPLSm1 has been possible and a consensus sequence has been obtained. Interestingly, an unusual structural motif of this N-glycan structure, has also been characterized in *L. stagnalis* (24).

Although the chemical synthesis of this glycan epitope remains a possibility, it is far from certain that its use in a vaccine is a viable possibility given the problem of blocking antibody production. This is particularly the case since the presence of antibodies to *S. mansoni* carbohydrate epitopes is strongly correlated to a state of non-resistance to reinfection in human populations (16). Further efforts at characterizing and producing protective molecules have, therefore, concentrated on protein antigens and in particular molecules secreted or excreted by schistosomula, but nevertheless present in adult worms. The reason for the latter is that adult worms constitute the major source of antigenic stimulus during infection and maintain the immune response that prevents reinfection, a phenomenon known as concomitant immunity (25).

Naturally, there is no reason why such molecules should not be present on the surface of schistosomula and several groups have set out to clone the protein parts of surface glycoproteins. One such approach is based on the observation that in the mouse model protective antibodies are in fact directed against the protein moieties of surface antigens (26). Up till now, the only published example of a cloned schistosomulum surface membrane antigen is that of a 18 kD protein (27). However, no data exists as to its protective value.

Excretory-Secretory Antigens In Protection

Two separate approaches led us to the molecular cloning of non-surface protective protein antigens. The first was the demonstration of the primordial importance of antigens excreted and secreted by schistosomula (schistosomula released products : SRP-A) in the induction of a protective IgE response in the rat and in primates. The second element was a pragmatic approach based on the search for protein antigens common to infective larvae and adult worms. SRP-A induces the production of IgE antibodies that are cytotoxic for schistosomula in the presence of macrophages, eosinophils or platelets and that transfer immunity to naive rats against a challenge infection (28). Direct immunization with SRP-A also protects rats to a large extent against infection. The IgE present in anti-SRP-A sera recognized two major antigens at 22 and 26 kD along with other minor bands. Interestingly, an IgE monoclonal antibody that reproduced the cytotoxic and protective properties of anti-SRP-A IgE also recognized a 26 kD antigen (14). In contrast, anti-SRP-A IgG antibodies recognized the same range of schistosomulum surface antigens as infection serum, as well as a protein of about 29 kD present in the in vitro translation products of adult worm mRNA (29).

Molecular Cloning Of The P28-I Antigen

The definition of a 28 kD molecule (P28-I) as a major protective antigen derived from the second element of the approach that aimed at developing polyclonal, monospecific antibody probes for screening cDNA libraries (30). Sera were raised in rats against a series of fractions of adult worm proteins separated on SDS-polyacrylamide gels. Of the fractions tested only one, against a 28 kDa band, produced antibodies that recognized both an in vitro translation product of adult worm mRNA, and a ^{125}I-labelled schistosomulum surface protein, albeit weakly. The anti-P28 serum was highly cytotoxic for schistosomula in the presence of eosinophils and this was demonstrably due to the IgG2a antibody subclass. Both passive transfer of the anti-P28 sera, and direct immunization with the electroeluted P28 fraction was extremely protective against a challenge infection in rats (65-70 %) and mice (43%) (31). In addition, helper T cell lines were developed against the P28 fraction (32) and their passive transfer protected rats against infection (85%). This protection was related to early production of anti-P28 antibodies.

The major protective element of the P28 fraction, P28-I was cloned from an adult worm cDNA expression library in the vector lambda gt11 (33). Three independent clones were actually cloned and sequenced. The full length sequence was obtained by rescreening the library with an oligonucleotide probe derived from the 5' end of the longest insert. Two more candidates were obtained and all five clones contained overlapping sequences corresponding to a 28 kD protein of 211 aminoacids and was termed P28-I. The sequence was confirmed by the sequences of two tryptic peptides obtained from the native protein.

The recombinant protein was initially expressed in E. coli as a fusion protein with the first eleven aminoacids of the lambda phage CII protein. The protein was highly immunogenic and induced the production of antibodies specific for the native protein and cytotoxic for schistosomula in the presence of eosinophils. Initial studies showed that direct immunization of rats and hamsters induced levels of protection of 65 and 50 % respectively.

Preliminary experiments using baboons immunized with E. coli produced P28-I also indicated that the recombinant antigen protected against a challenge infection although wide individual variations in response were noted (34). It was notable, however, that the mean granuloma size in immunized animals was reduced, indicating a possible reduction in egg-induced pathology.

A subsequent experiment confirmed both aspects of protection in baboons. Of three groups of six animals immunized with different dose regimes of P28-I in the presence of aluminium hydroxide one group receiving three doses of 67 µg of recombinant P28-I were protected at a mean level of 38 %, with individual variations from 25-80 % (Boulanger *et al.*, manuscript in preparation). A second group of animals having received two doses of 100 μg, paradoxically showed no overall reduction in worm burden. However, these animals had fewer granulomatous lesions and the latter were smaller in size than in controls. In this case, both egg production and the granuloma reaction were reduced. These effects have subsequently been reproduced in the mouse model (I. Wolowczuk, unpublished observations).

More recent studies using rats and mice have shown that multiple doses of P28-I are not necessary to induce protection. On the contrary, single doses of P28-I with either aluminium hydroxide or BCG as adjuvant protect rats and mice significantly against infection (Grezel *et al.*, manuscript in preparation). This is an encouraging result in the context of human vaccination where repeated doses may be difficult or impossible to administer effectively. These results are highly promising in that P28-I seems to fulfill the requirements for a candidate vaccine. However the major remaining problems concern the variability in the immune response to P28-I and its possible MHC restriction, and the fact that overall protection levels in primates are not adequate to justify human trials.

Epitopic Characteristics Of P28-I

In order to study the major epitopes of P28-I for both T and B cell responses the primary sequence was analyzed for exposed sequences and for mobility and accessibility. Peptide fragments corresponding to these criteria were synthesized and tested for their capacity to restimulate T cells from infected or immunized animals, and their recognition by antibodies. Three peptides were thus tested and two (aminoacids 24-43 and 115-131) were found to contain major epitopes for IgG antibodies in the rat, but not for IgE (35). The antibodies raised against the 24-43 peptide were of the IgG2a subclass, were cytotoxic in vitro for schistosomula and recognized the native P28-I antigen. The same 24-43 peptide, as well as the 140-153 peptide also contained major T cell epitopes. T cell lines specific for the 24-43 peptide when passively transferred to rats immunized with P28-I led to a significant increase in specific IgE.

The MHC restriction of the response to P28-I was tested using both recombinant antigen and synthetic peptides in the mouse model (36). A preliminary survey using H-2 congenic mice on a BALB background showed that the P28-I response was indeed under MHC control and that the H-2^b haplotype determined a low response to P28-I and its peptides, whilst H-2^d and H-2^k haplotypes determined high responders.

A further feature of the mouse immune response to P28-I was that resistance to infection could be transferred by T helper cell lines from BALB/c mice immunized with the recombinant antigen, but not by the corresponding immune sera. This result confirms observation made in the mouse model using other antigen preparations (37).

The humoral responses toward P28-I and its peptides of human subjects after oxamniquine treatment, that have been defined as either susceptible or resistant to reinfection has also been examined (38). The main feature of the response toward the whole recombinant antigen was a significant increase in the IgG4 response after treatment in the susceptible population. Two of the peptides (115-131 and 140-153) contained epitopes recognized by IgE antibodies, and this response increased after treatment in both susceptible and resistant individuals. Use of the peptides also showed that specific IgG1 antibodies were produced by the immune population after treatment, whereas the susceptible population was again characterized by a strong production of IgG4 antibodies. While the implications for a vaccination programme using recombinant P28-I are difficult to assess, the results do indicate that manipulation of the immune response may be possible in order to favour a protective response. Taken together the results in experimental animals and in humans also suggest that a synthetic vaccine based on peptides 115-131 and 140-153 may be a viable prospect.

P28-I Is A Glutathione-S-Transferase

The aminoacid sequence of P28-I over much of its length displays a low level of homology to rat glutathione-S-transferase (GSH transferases) of class α and class μ, but not of class π (39). However, high levels of homology to class α or μ subunits occur over short regions of the aminoacid sequence. Recombinant P28-I produced in either yeast or *E. coli* possesses GSH-transferase activity and when native GSH-transferase was purified by affinity chromatography from adult worms, and subjected to sequence analysis, the latter was found identical to that of the cloned molecule. No significant level of homology was found to the 26 kD GSH-transferase previously cloned and sequenced from *S. japonicum* (40). One consequence of this finding was that it was now possible to purify recombinant P28-I to homogeneity by a single step purification involving passage over a glutathione-agarose affinity column. This largely obviates problems of contamination due to *E. coli* components and particularly LPS and endotoxin. A second possible consequence was an eventual cross-reactivity with the mammalian enzyme. This has never been detected whatever the technique used, however.

We had previously characterized P28-I as a schistosomulum surface protein, however electron microscopy using the immunogold technique demonstrated that although the antigen is present in the adult worm tegument, protonephridial cells and subtegumental parenchymal cells, it is not exposed on the surface. The antigen is also present in the tegument of schistosomula, and also in the head gland from which tegumental components may be derived. The latter location may explain a transient surface exposure. Neither the aminoacid sequence, nor the function of the molecule are consistent with its being an integral membrane protein.

The function of GSH transferases may be consistent with a role in the defence of the parasite against the immune defences in the host. The fatty acid hydroperoxide-GSH peroxidase and GSH transferase activities expressed by P28-I indicate a possible involvement in inhibiting lipid peroxidation and scavenging hydroxyalkenals produced by the release of highly reactive oxygen species by effector cells. It is thus tempting to speculate that an effective immune response directed against the enzyme may act in part by neutralizing this defensive enzyme.

Other Cloned Antigens: Prospects For A Composite Vaccine

The problem of MHC restriction of the immune response may indicate that a single antigen vaccine against schistosomiasis will not be adequate. This is not necessarily the case since the use of different adjuvants and dosing schedules, and the selection of epitopes using synthetic peptides could well obviate the necessity for antigen cocktails.

At the present time, only two other antigens known to protect against schistosome infections have been cloned. One is the *S. japonicum* 26 kD GSH-transferase (40) previously mentioned. It is indeed interesting that two of the protective antigens should possess the same enzyme activity although they belong to different gene families. This underlines the crucial role played by GSH-transferases in the survival of the parasite. Cross-reactivity exists between P28-I and 28 kD molecules in other species of schistosome, including *S. japonicum*, but it remains to be seen whether the interspecific antigenic community is sufficient to permit cross-species protection.

A major target of the cell-mediated immunity developed in the mouse model after immunization with *S. mansoni* adult-worm antigens in the presence of BCG is a 97 kD molecule (41). This turned out to be paramyosin, an invertebrate muscle protein involved in the 'catch' mechanism of muscle contraction (42). Purified native paramyosin or the ß-galactosidase fusion protein both protected mice against infection by intradermal vaccination in the presence of BCG. Paramyosin is not uniquely a target of cell-mediated immunity since it is a major allergen in rat infections, and is also recognized by IgE in some human infection sera (43).

A large variety of schistosome antigens have now been cloned, some of which may be candidate vaccines, including a 50 kD schistosomulum surface antigen (44) and a cercarial esterase (45). However, their potential remains to be demonstrated in animal models.

The main prospect for a composite vaccine at the moment could be the combination of P28-I with paramyosin and work along these lines is in progress.

CONCLUSIONS

The prospects for an effective vaccine against *S. mansoni* are very real. The recombinant P28-I antigen is a candidate molecule for such a vaccine. Although high levels of protection can be induced by single doses of P28-I, it remains likely that MHC restriction of the immune response in outbred populations will necessitate either a manipulation of the immune response by selective epitopic presentation, or the incorporation of other protective antigens in the definitive vaccine. Several candidates for a vaccine cocktail have been cloned, one of which is paramyosin. However, further work remains to be accomplished, notably on the effects of vaccinating children previously exposed to schistosome antigens in utero, and on the possibility of vaccinating individuals after chemotherapy to eliminate an ongoing infection. Indeed, such a combination of chemotherapy with a vaccine strategy could well be the main hope for control of schistosomiasis.

REFERENCES

1. Prescott, N. M. (1987): *Parasitology Today* 3:21-24.
2. Coles, G. C., Bruce, J. I., Kinoti, G. K., Mutahi, W. T., Dias, L. C. S., Rocha, R. S., and Katz, N. (1987): *Parasitology Today* 3:349-350.
3. Phillips, S. M., Colley, D. G. (1978): *Prog. Allergy* 24:49-182.
4. Capron, A., Dessaint, J. P., Capron, M., Ouma, A., and Butterworth, A. E. (1987): *Science* 238:1065-1072.
5. Sher, A., Hieny, S., James, S. L., and Asofsky, R. (1982): *J. Immunol.* 128:1880-1884.
6. Pearce, E. J., and James, S. L. (1986): *Parasite Immunol.* 8:513-527.
7. Harn, D., Quinn, J. J., Ciarci, C. M., and Ko, A. I. (1987): *J. Immunol.* 138:1571-1580.
8. Ward, R. E. M., and McLaren, D. J. (1988): *Parasitology* 96:63-84.
9. Bickle, Q. D., and Ford, M. J. (1982): *J. Immunol.* 125:2101-2106.
10. Capron, M., and Capron, A. (1986): *Parasitology Today* 2:69-72.
11. Capron, M., Nogueira-Queiroz, J. A., Papin, J. P., and Capron, A. (1984): *Cell Immunol.* 83:60-72.

12. Joseph, M., Auriault, C., Capron, A., Vorng, H., and Viens, P. (1983): *Nature* 303:8100-812.
13. Grzych, J. M., Capron, M., Bazin, H., and Capron, A. (1982): *J. Immunol.* 129:2739-2743.
14. Verwaerde, C., Joseph, M., Capron, M., Pierce, R. J., Damonneville, M., Velge, F., Auriault, C., and Capron, A. (1987): *J. Immunol.* 138:4441-4446.
15. Khalife, J., Capron, M., Capron, A., Grzych, J. M., Butterworth, A. E., Dunne, D. W., Ouma, J. M. (1986): *J. Exp. Med.* 164:1626-1640.
16. Butterworth, A. E., Bensted-Smith, R., Capron, A., Capron, M., Dalton, P. R., Dunne, D. W., Grzych, J. M., Kaikuri, H. C., Khalife, J., Liech, D., Mugambi, M., Ouma, J. M., Arap Siogok, T. K., and Sturrock, R. F. (1987): *Parasitology* 94:281-300.
17. Dissous, C., Dissous, C., and Capron, A. (1981): *Mol. Biochem. Parasitol.* 3:215-225.
18. Dissous, C., Grzych, J. M., and Capron, A. (1982): *J. Immunol.* 129:2232-2234.
19. Dissous, C., Grzych, J. M., and Capron, A. (1985): *Mol. Biochem. Parasitol.* 16:277-288.
20. Grzych, J. M., Capron, M., and Capron, A. (1984): *J. Immunol.* 133:998-1004.
21. Grzych, J. M., Capron, M., Lambert, P. H., Dissous, C., Torres, S., and Capron, A. (1985): *Nature* 316:74-75.
22. Grzych, J. M., Dissous, C., Capron, M., Torres, S., Lambert, P. H., and Capron, A. (1987): *J. Exp. Med.* 165:865-878.
23. Dissous, C., Grzych, J. M., and Capron, A. (1986): *Nature* 323:443-445.
24. Van Kuik, J. A., Sijbesma, R. P., Kamerling, J. P., Vliegenthardt, J. F. G., and Wood, E. J. (1987): In: Proceedings of the 9th International Symposium, *Glycoconjugates,* edited by J. Montreuil, A. Verbert, G. Spik, and B. Fournet, Abstr. A-89. A. Lerouge, Tourcoing (France).
25. Smithers, S. R., Terry, R. J. (1967): *Trans. R. Soc. Trop. Med. Hyg.* 61:517.
26. Omer-Ali, P., Magee, A. I., Kelly, C., and Simpson, A. J. G. (1986): *J. Immunol.* 137:3601-3607.
27. Dalton, J. P., Tom, T. D., and Strand, M. (1987): *J. Immunol.* 84:4268-4272.
28. Damonneville, M., Auriault, C., Verwaerde, C., Delannoye, A., Pierce, R. J., and Capron, A. (1986): *Clin. exp. Immunol.* 65:244-252.
29. Pierce, R. J., Aimar, C., Balloul, J. M., Delarue, M., Grausz, D., Verwaerde, C., and Capron, A. (1985): *Mol. Biochem. Parasitol.* 15:171-188.
30. Balloul, J. M., Pierce, R. J., Grzych, J. M., and Capron, A. (1985): *Mol. Biochem. Parasitol.* 17:105-114.
31. Balloul, J. M., Grzych, J. M., Pierce, R. J., Delannoye, A., Damonneville, M., and Capron, A. (1987): *J. Immunol.* 138:3448-3453.
32. Auriault, C., Balloul, J. M., Pierce, R. J., Delannoye, A., Damonneville, M., and Capron, A. (1987): *Infect. Immun.* 55:1163-1169.
33. Balloul, J. M., Sondermeyer, P., Dreyer, D., Capron, M., Grzych, J. M., Pierce, R. J., Carvallo, D., Lecocq, J. P., and Capron, A. (1987): *Nature* 326:149-153.
34. Balloul, J. M., Boulanger, D., Sondermeyer, P., Dreyer, D., Capron, M., Grzych, J. M., Pierce, R. J., Carvallo, D., Lecocq, J. P., and Capron, A. (1987): In: *Molecular Paradigms for the Eradication of Helminth Parasites,* edited by A. MacInnes, pp. 77-84. Alan R. Liss, New York.
35. Auriault, C., Gras-Masse, H., Wolowczuk, I., Pierce, R. J., Balloul, J. M., Neyrinck, J. L., Drobecq, H., Tartar, A., and Capron, A. (1988): *J. Immunol.* 141:1687-1694.
36. Wolowczuk, I., Auriault, C., Gras-Masse, H., Vendeville, C., Balloul, J. M., Tartar, A., and Capron, A. (1989): *J. Immunol.* 142:1342-1350.
37. James, S. L., and Sher, A. (1986): *Parasitology Today* 2:134-137.
38. Auriault, C., Gras-Masse, H., Capron, M., Butterworth, A. E., Balloul, J. M., Pierce, R. J., Neyrinck, J. L., Tartar, A., and Capron, A. (1989): (Submitted for Publication).
39. Taylor, J. B., Vidal, A., Torpier, G., Meyer, D. J., Roitsch, C., Balloul, J. M., Southan, C., Sondermeyer, P., Remble, S., Lecocq, J. P., Capron, A., and Ketterer, B. (1980): *EMBO J.* 7:465-472.
40. Smith, D. B., Davern, K. M., Board, P. G., Tiu, W. U., Garcia, E. G., Mitchell, G. F. (1986): *Proc. Natl. Acad. Sci.* 83:8703-8707.

41. Pearce, E. J., James, S. L., Dalton, J., Barrall, A., Ramos, C., Strand, M., and Sher, A. (1986): *J. Immunol.* 137:3593-3600.
42. Lanar, D. E., Pearce, E. J., James, S. L., and Sher, A. (1986): *Science* 234 : 593-596.
43. Boutin, P., Pierce, R. J., Lepresle, T., and Capron, A. (1989): (Submitted for Publication).
44. Havercroft, J. C., Huggins, M. C., Nene, V., Dunne, D. W., Richardson, B. A., Taylor, D. W., and Butterworth, A. E. (1988): *Mol. Biochem. Parasitol.* 30:83-88.
45. Newport, G. R., McKerrow, J. H., Hedstrom, R,, Petitt, M., McGarrigle, L., Barr, P. J., and Agabian, N. (1988): *J. Biol. Chem.* 263:12179-13184.

Molecular Aspects of Immune Response and Infectious Diseases, edited by H. Kiyono, E. Jirillo, and C. DeSimone. Raven Press, Ltd., New York, © 1990.

2 2

Potential Utilization of Idiotype Vaccines to Induce Influenza Virus Immunity

C. A. Bona and J. L. Schulman

Department of Microbiology, Mount Sinai School of Medicine New York, New York, USA

INTRODUCTION

The lack of success in developing vaccines able to elicit long lasting crossreactive immunity against influenza viruses is related to the unusual capacity of the virus for significant antigenic variation. Two genetic mechanisms are responsible for this phenomenon: a) antigenic shift which results from periodic genetic reassortment of human and animal influenza viruses; and b) antigenic drift which results from stepwise selection of antigenic variants in nature. As antigenically new strains emerge as a consequence of one of these two mechanisms, immunization with older strains is no longer effective. These observations have stimulated investigators to explore new approaches for the development of vaccines against influenza viruses endowed with the ability to elicit long lasting crossreactive immunity. Among these new approaches the use of idiotype vaccine is one of the most attractive since, in principle, an Ab2β - anti-idiotype antibody carrying the internal image of hemagglutinin (HA) or neuraminidase (NA) can activate clones producing antibodies against various influenza virus subtypes.

The rationale of this approach is based on a) demonstration that antibodies specific for HA or NA of various influenza virus subtypes bear crossreactive idiotypes and, therefore, such clones can be activated by the same anti-idiotype antibody and b) the Ab2β of HA or NA, mimics the respective epitopes and, therefore, can stimulate clones which produce antibodies against various influenza virus subtypes or variants of the same subtype.

INDUCTION OF ANTI-INFLUENZA VIRUS IMMUNITY BY AB2

There are numerous reports demonstrating that the Ab2β can stimulate host immunity against bacterial viral and parasitic antigens, as well against tumor cells (1) (see also Chapter 20 by Eichmann). In contrast, there is limited information with respect to the induction of anti-HA or NA immune responses by anti-idiotype (Id) antibodies.

Moran, et al., (2), prepared several syngeneic monoclonal antibodies which recognize a crossreactive idiotype was demonstrable in sera of mice immunized with influenza A viruses of different subtypes. However, adsorption of such sera on anti-idiotype columns did not significantly deplete anti-viral antibody indicating that Id+ antibody was only a minor component of the anti-viral response (3). In addition, Id+ antibodies could be detected in sera of human subjects following immunization with trivalent influenza virus vaccine (4). The structural basis for this IdX was identified by Western blotting using one of these monoclonal Ab2 (SP3-5A) demonstrated binding only to the heavy chains of Id+ antibodies. On the basis of these observations of a crossreactive idiotype on monoclonal antibodies specific for H3 and H1 hemagglutinins, the expression of this idiotype in sera of mice immunized with different influenza viruses and evidence that the idiotope was expressed among different species, we speculated that immunization with monoclonal anti-idiotype theoretically might generate or prime for crossreactive anti-influenza responses.

In the first attempts to use idiotype vaccines against influenza, we investigated the priming effects of anti-idiotype immunization on hemagglutinating inhibiting (HI) responses following challenge with PR8 (H1N1) or X-31 (H3N2) viruses. We employed two other monoclonal anti-PY206 antibodies (SN3-1A and SN3-9A) in doses ranging from 0.1 to 5 μg/mouse, and included IDA-10 (A48Id) as a control. At the doses tested, anti-idiotype immunization had no effect on HI response following PR8 or X-31 challenge. Similarly, anti-idiotype immunization had no effect on HI antibody responses when virus challenge took place 21 days instead of 14 days after immunization.

In the next group of experiments, the effects of two immunizations of BALB/c mice with different doses of SP3-5A were compared to the priming effects of primary immunization with virus. There was no priming for an X-31-specific HI response at any of the doses of SP3-5A tested. In contrast, two immunization with 5 μg of SP3-5A appeared to prime for a 2° anti-PR8 response 7 and 21 days after challenge almost as effectively as 1° immunization with PR8 virus.

A comparable priming effect on PR8 but not on X-31 responses was observed when C3H mice were primed with two injections of 5 μg of SP3-5A. In view of previous reports indicating that the effects of anti-idiotype immunization may be enhanced when the anti-Id is coupled to a carrier, we assayed the effects of two different doses of SP3-5A coupled to KLH. Two injections of SP3-5A-KLH conjugates (5 or 10 μg each) had no effect on HI antibody responses following either PR8 or X-31 virus challenge (data not shown).

In other experiments, the effects of anti-idiotype immunization on aerosol infection of mice with PR8 or X-31 viruses were assayed. With either virus there were no differences between anti-Id immunization mice and controls in terms of pulmonary virus titers, lung lesions or HI antibody responses following infection.

In summary, we employed a syngeneic monoclonal anti-idiotype antibody which theoretically possessed ideal attributes for a candidate idiotype vaccine: recognition of an interspecies crossreactive antibody; reactivity with antibody specific for different influenza A virus hemagglutinins and specificity for a variable region structure on the heavy chain. Nevertheless, at best, our results demonstrate only a marginal effect in priming for anti-PR8 responses and no effect of anti-idiotype immunization on virus infection (3).

It is possible that in view of the heterogeneity of anti-HA antibodies, stimulation of a particular Id by an Ab2β may not be expected to significantly alter the total anti-viral response. Alternatively, the absence of appropriate syngeneic helper effect may be responsible.

Recently, Anders *et al.* (5) raised polyclonal rabbit anti-Id antibodies against mAbs specific for various epitopes of HA or H1N1 Mempis 71H-Bel N (H3N1) virus. Rabbit anti-Id antibodies were directed against an IdI of mAbs specific for HA. Immunization of mice with two of these rabbit anti-Id antibodies induced anti-HA responses with neutralizing activity. In addition, analysis of serum antibodies from these mice revealed additional distinct subsets of antibodies which bound not only to H3 but also to H1 or H2 viruses. Since the induction of antibodies to HA of different subtypes is not observed in antibody responses elicited subsequent to viral immunization, these data clearly show that the Ab2 can induce crossreactive immunity against viruses of various subtypes.

Mayer *et al.* (6) studied the effect of a syngeneic monoclonal anti-Id antibody (RM1) which recognizes an IdX shared by N1 and N2 specific antibodies designated as Py203 IdX. Py203-Id is a marker of a large fraction of anti-NA clones. The adsorption of sera obtained from animals injected with influenza viruses on corresponding recombinant viruses and RM1 indicate that a significant fraction of NA-specific Abs express the Py203-Id. However, this Id certainly is also expressed on Ig molecules devoid of anti-NA activity (parallel set). The clones expressing this Id can be expanded by two injections of the monoclonal anti-Id Ab RM1. Priming of BALB/c mice with minute amounts of RM1 followed two weeks later by a boost with the same amount of Ab caused a significant increase of Py203-Id bearing immunoglobulins without a parallel expansion of anti-NA Ab producing cells. In contrast, priming with RM1 followed by immunization with influenza-A virus induced an increase in both PY203-Id$^+$ and NA-specific responses.

Since this monoclonal anti-Id antibody was able to prime NA-specific clones but not to cause their differentiation to plasma cells, one may consider this antibody as an Ab2β. The priming effect of Ab2β is related to the binding of anti-Id Abs to a complementary Id expressed on the Ig receptor of clones with various antigenic specificities. This study demonstrates that an anti-Id Ab can function in the activation of clones producing protective Abs without acting as the internal image of the antigen involved.

STUDY OF THE EXPRESSION OF CROSSREACTIVE IDIOTYPE ON MONOCLONAL ANTIBODIES SPECIFIC FOR PR8 SEQUENTIAL LABORATORY VARIANTS

The data summarized above suggest that it is possible to stimulate antibody responses against major influenza virus glycoproteins HA and NA by anti-Id antibodies. Therefore, it was important to investigate whether antibodies specific for influenza virus variants are related and particularly if they share a crossreactive idiotype which can be target of regulatory effect of Ab2α or Ab2β.

We generated four monoclonal antibodies specific for an identical or closely related topographic region on HA1 of sequential virus variants. Sequence analysis of the HA genes of these variants revealed that their reciprocal binding patterns were attributable to substitutions of nucleotide 555 in the SA region of HA1 (7).

In addition to their closely related antigen specificity, three of the four antibodies shared a crossreactive idiotype. To obtain further insight into the structural basis of their related paratopes and the IdX, variable regions of the heavy and light chains were sequenced. The results revealed that primary structures were quite different, documenting that a variety of antibody structures are capable of reacting with subtly different structures in biologically imported antigens.

For example, Py102, the antibody specific for PR8 HA is encoded by a V_H gene derived from V_H 7183 family, associated with a D gene FL16.2 and J_H4 and V_K8 associated to J_K5. VH113 sharing Py102 IdX and specific for first sequential variant uses a V_H gene from J558 family in association with SP2-6 D segment and J_H1 and V_K10 associated with J_K2. VM202 antibody specific for second sequential variant which also shared PY102 IdX uses a gene from V_H 7183 and a V_K2 in association with J_K5 (7). These results suggest that similar contacting residues involved in idiotype-anti-idiotype interactions can be borne by variable regions encoded by various V_H or V_K genes.

The presence of crossreactive idiotypes on antibodies specific for wild-type virus and its variants suggest that clones producing such IdX or alternatively by anti-Id antibodies carrying the internal image of the antigen. Our present efforts are directed towards rising polyclonal rabbit anti-Id antibodies as immunogens. Our rationale is as follows: a) we already have evidence that some of these rabbit antisera detect a crossreactive idiotype(s); b) because of their polyclonal nature, there is greater likelihood that some of the rabbit anti-Ids may be Ab2β and, hence, bear an internal image capable of eliciting a crossreactive anti-HA response.

REFERENCES

1. Bona, C., editor (1988): *Biological Applications of Antiidiotypes*, Vol. II. CRC Press, Boca Raton, Florida.
2. Moran, T., Liu, Y. -N. C., Schulman, J. L., and Bona, C. A. (1984): *Proc. Natl. Acad. Sci. USA* 81:1809-1812.
3. Moran, M. T., Reale, M. A., Monestier, M., Mayer, R., Schulman, J. L., and Bona, C. A. (1986): *Concepts Immunopathol.* 3:233-252.
4. Sigal, N. H., Chan, M., Reale, M. A., Moran, T., Beilin, Y., Schulman, J. L., and Bona, C. (1987): *J. Immunol.* 139:1985-1990.
5. Anders, E. M., Kapaklis-Deliyannis, G. P., and White, D. O. (1990): *J. Virol.* 63:2758-2767.
6. Mayer, R., Ioannides, C., Moran, T., Johansson, B., and Bona, C. (1987): *Virol. Imm.* 1:121-134.
7. Meek, K., Johansson, B., Schulman, J., Bona, C., and Capra, J. D. (1989): *Proc. Natl. Acad. Sci.* 86:4664-4668.

Index